**Current
Psychiatric
Therapies
Vol. 12 — 1972**

AN ANNUAL PUBLICATION

Vol. 12 – 1972

Current

Psychiatric

Therapies

Edited by

Jules H. Masserman,
M.D.

Professor of Psychiatry
and Neurology
Northwestern University
Chicago, Illinois

GRUNE & STRATTON

NEW YORK • LONDON

Grune & Stratton, Inc.
111 Fifth Avenue
New York, New York 10003

Library of Congress Catalog Card Number 61-9411

International Standard Book Number 0-8089-0765-4

Printed in the United States of America

Published annually and available in print:
Vols. 1-11

dated consecutively 1961-1971

Table of Contents

PART I: Childhood and Adolescence

PART II: Adult Psychotherapeutic Techniques

PART III: Psychopharmacology and Physical Modalities

PART VII: The Aged

PART VIII: Contributions from Abroad

Preface

It has been my perennial purpose as editor to keep these volumes abreast of advances in as many aspects of psychiatric theory and therapy as possible. A retrospective glance at successive degrees of interest in the special fields reflected in the 12 issues of the series since 1960 reveals these significant variations:

A marked increase in concern about "primary prevention," i.e., the amelioration of poverty, overcrowding, ignorance, physical disease, and other presumed direct or indirect causes of disorders of behavior.

A corresponding concentration on problems of childhood and adolescence.

A diversification of adult dyadic therapies, with classically stereotyped psychoanalytic techniques giving place to more directly goal-oriented, versatile, briefer, and operationally effective methods.

An increasing interest in group therapies, ranging in focus from the nuclear family to wider "systems approaches" comprising extensive kinship, educational, neighborhood, industrial, and other transactional relationships.

An exploration of new and sometimes daring procedures in these fields, from brief "training" episodes through cathartic "sensitivity" sessions to prolonged and searchingly protracted "marathons."

A peaking of interest in psychopharmacology about midway in the series, succeeded by chapters in later issues advocating greater restraint in the use of medication and more conservative expectations as to lasting therapeutic effects.

Reevaluations of "community psychiatry," with growing doubts as to the usefulness of many "mental health centers" unless they developed special programs for limited objectives such as help for unwed mothers, the legalized supervision and therapy of alcohol and drug addictions, the rehabilitation of patients discharged from psychiatric hospitals, and other such endeavors.

An increasing appreciation of relevant progress in other countries, including those with contrasting economic and political systems.

A concurrent rejection of doctrinaire rigidity in psychiatric theory and practice, a salutary tendency toward more culturally as well as biologically and experientially contingent formulations as to human behavior and its vicissitudes, and a concern that young psychiatrists be accordingly trained more broadly and comprehensively.

Finally, a growing and editorially welcome, though still incomplete, aversion to jargon, ambiguity, and prolixity in psychiatric writing in favor of greater brevity, clarity, and cogency of style.

By thus reflecting current and future advances in psychiatric thought and therapy as reported by leading specialists in various fields—to whom the editor is perennially indebted—I trust that this and succeeding volumes will continue to deserve the worldwide readership they have received.

Jules H. Masserman, M.D.

Northwestern University
January 1, 1972

Roster of Contributors

Abroms, Gene M., M.D., Associate Professor of Psychiatry, University of Wisconsin Medical School, Madison, Wisconsin.

Altshuler, Kenneth Z., M.D., Associate Clinical Professor of Psychiatry, College of Physicians and Surgeons, Columbia University, New York, New York.

Ban, Thomas A., M.D., Associate Professor and Director, Division of Psychopharmacology, Department of Psychiatry, McGill University, Montreal, P.Q., Canada.

Barish, Julian I., M.D., President, Society for Adolescent Psychiatry of New York, Larchmont, New York.

Beyel, Virginia, R.N., Central Islip State Hospital, Central Islip, New York.

Blachly, Paul H., M.D., Professor of Psychiatry, University of Oregon Medical School, Portland, Oregon.

Chappel, John N., M.D., Assistant Professor of Psychiatry, Division of Biological Sciences, University of Chicago, Chicago, Illinois.

Clancy, Helen G., Ph.D., Senior Research Fellow, Department of Child Health, University of Queensland, Brisbane, Australia.

Daniels, Robert S., M.D., Professor and Director, Department of Psychiatry, University of Cincinnati, Cincinnati, Ohio.

Fiorentino, Diane, B.A., Central Islip State Hospital, Central Islip, New York.

Fracchia, John, M.A., Central Islip State Hospital, Central Islip, New York.

Freundlich, David, M.D., Director, Manhattan Center for the Whole Person, New York, New York.

Gendzel, Ivan B., M.D., Clinical Assistant Professor of Psychiatry, Stanford University School of Medicine, Palo Alto, California.

Glasser, William, M.D., Institute for Reality Therapy, Los Angeles, California.

Greene, Bernard L., M.D., Clinical Professor of Psychiatry, Abraham Lincoln School of Medicine, University of Illinois, Chicago, Illinois.

Harlan, William L., M.D., Associate Professor, Department of Preventive Medicine and Public Health, Creighton University School of Medicine, Omaha, Nebraska.

Heller, Abraham, M.D., Director, Comprehensive Community Mental Health Center, Denver General Hospital, Denver, Colorado.

Herschelman, Philip, M.D., Fellow in Psychiatry, Chestnut Lodge, Rockville, Maryland.

Hiatt, Harold, M.D., Associate Professor of Psychiatry, University of Cincinnati College of Medicine, and Chief, Psychiatry Service, Veterans Administration Hospital, Cincinnati, Ohio.

Hollister, Leo E., M.D., Medical Investigator, Veterans Administration Hospital, Palo Alto, California, and Associate Professor of Medicine, Stanford University School of Medicine, Stanford, California.

Karpman, Stephen B., M.D., Group Therapist, Eric Berne Institute, San Francisco, California.

Lehmann, Heinz E., M.D., Professor and Chairman, Department of Psychiatry, McGill University, Montreal, P.Q., Canada.

Lipowski, Z. J., M.D., Professor of Psychiatry, Dartmouth Medical School, Hanover, New Hampshire.

López Ibor, Juan J., M.D., Professor of Psychiatry and Psychological Medicine, University of Madrid, Madrid, Spain.

Lynch, Henry T., M.D., Professor and Chairman, Department of Preventive Medicine and Public Health, Creighton University School of Medicine, Omaha, Nebraska.

McBride, Glen, Ph.D., Reader, Animal Behaviour Unit, Psychology Department, University of Queensland, Brisbane, Australia.

McConaghy, Neil, M.D., D.P.M., Associate Professor of Psychiatry, University of New South Wales, Sidney, Australia.

McGee, Thomas F., Ph.D., Director, Mental Health Division, Chicago Board of Health, Chicago, Illinois.

Meldman, Monte J., M.D., Director of Research, Forest Hospital, Des Plaines, Illinois.

Merlis, Sidney, M.D., Director of Psychiatric Research, Central Islip State Hospital, Central Islip, New York.

Musser, Marc J., M.D., Chief Medical Director, Veterans Administration, Department of Medicine and Surgery, Washington, D.C.

Novick, Rudolph G., M.D., Clinical Director, Forest Hospital, Des Plaines, Illinois.

Ostrowski, M.V., M.A., Staff, Forest Hospital, Des Plaines, Illinois.

Polak, Paul, M.D., Director, Southwest Denver Community Mental Health Services, Inc., Denver, Colorado.

Rainer, John D., M.D., Associate Professor of Clinical Psychiatry, College of Physicians and Surgeons, Columbia University, New York, New York.

Reidda, Phil, M.S., Coordinator of Research and Evaluation, Mental Health Division, Chicago Board of Health, Chicago, Illinois.

Rosenthal, Saul H., M.D., Associate Professor of Psychiatry, University of Texas Medical School, San Antonio, Texas.

Schonfeld, William A., M.D., Deceased.

Sheppard, Charles, M.A., Central Islip State Hospital, Central Islip, New York.

Squire, Morris B., B.A., Director, Forest Hospital, Des Plaines, Illinois.

Stein, Calvert, M.D., Psychiatrist, Springfield, Massachusetts.

Steinberg, Fannie, M.S.W., Acting Director, Division of Social Services, New York City Housing Authority, New York, New York.

Sussman, Robert B., M.D., Formerly Director of Psychiatry (Housing), New York City Department of Mental Health and Mental Retardation Services; Clinical Director, Four Winds Hospital, Katonah, New York.

Walton, H. J., M.D., D.P.M., Senior Lecturer, Department of Psychiatry, University of Edinburgh, Edinburgh, Scotland.

Wells, Benjamin B., M.D., Deputy Chief Medical Director, Department of Medicine and Surgery, Veterans Administration, Washington, D.C.

Wolberg, Lewis R., M.D., Director, Center for Postgraduate Education, New York, N.Y.

Wolpe, Joseph, M.D., Professor of Psychiatry, Temple University Medical School and Eastern Pennsylvania Psychiatric Institute, Philadelphia, Pennsylvania.

Zunin, Leonard M., M.D., Director, Institute for Reality Therapy, Los Angeles, California.

CHILDHOOD AND ADOLESCENCE

Therapy of Childhood Autism in the Family

by Helen G. Clancy, Ph.D., and Glen McBride, Ph.D.

Diagnosis

Before discussing treatment it is essential to define the condition. The differential diagnosis of infantile autism usually constitutes a problem, because of the wide range of childhood disorders which involve behavior of a type commonly called "autistic." Elsewhere we have suggested that these are the usual behavioral responses to social isolation, which appear and develop whenever there is a deficiency in the infant-mother communication system, leading to the failure to develop a strong socializing bond (Clancy and McBride[6]). The resultant syndrome, the isolation syndrome, is present in institutionalized children, in family-reared but separated children, e.g., hospitalized children, and in families where the child's communicative abilities are impaired, e.g., by blindness, deafness, or mental deficiency, and, more insidiously, where the mother is inattentive to the infant for any reason, such as depression.

Again, the isolation syndrome is present when, for some reason as yet unexplained, the child rejects social contact and develops an autistic process within the mother-child relationship. By this we mean that a communicative system is established in which the child indicates preference for solitude and resists social intrusion and demands from others, and the family accommodates to his behavior and life-style. The autistic process leads to the isolation syndrome, but the clinical picture is differentiated from other disorders associated with the isolation syndrome by the following features:

    1. The use of "cutoff" behaviors by the child to establish and maintain isolation from others, specifically parents.

2. The absence of an effective bond between the child and another person, normally the mother. This lack of a bond may alternatively be expressed as absence of a stranger response by the child.

The four main categories of abnormal behavior to be seen in the isolation syndrome are:

1. Behavior indicating damage of perceptual functions; for example, the baby fails to give the normal orienting response to sources of stimulation, often sounds, or he may fail to respond communicatively to pain. These may equally be regarded as examples of inadequate socialization.
2. Behavior suggesting inappropriate communication within the mother-child interaction, for example, absence of the smiling response, eye contact, or cuddling.
3. Excessive use of self-stimulating behavior: rocking, knocking, spinning objects, or masturbation in older children. These also serve communicatively as cutoff behavior in the autistic process.
4. Varying degrees of functional retardation in skills, especially language, which depend on a socializing relationship with the mother. In the extreme case seen in the autistic process, the child resists all novelty in his personal routines and environment and characteristically rejects all but a very narrow range of foods.

The most serious diagnostic problem for the autistic process is the lack of efficient criteria for its detection in the first 12-18 months of life. For older children we use a screening test (see Appendix 1, Clancy et al.[3]) to detect cases for further diagnostic examination.

In the absence of known etiologies for the autistic process, our treatment is directed at the isolation syndrome and the self-isolating behavior. The treatment has also been used with success in other cases of the isolation syndrome within the age range of 1 to 7 years. Since the child becomes increasingly retarded in development with age, it seems important to begin treatment as early as possible.

The Unit of Treatment

Language and culture have profound effects on the concepts held and used in therapy. For example, we may look at a family as a group of individuals or a set of relationships. In exactly the same way, the disorder "infantile autism" can be seen as "an autistic child," emphasizing the individual, or it can be seen as "an autistic process within a family," emphasizing the behavioral basis of the relationships between individuals, with the abnormal behavior of the child reflecting these relationships. The consequences for therapy are profoundly different. One view leads to the treatment of an autistic child by a therapist, complemented by a social worker dealing with the family, i.e., two conventional roles; the other approach leads to the development of a team who share their specialist skills across conventional roles to develop a treatment program which is less fragmented than the traditional procedure.

We reject child-oriented treatment; though it can lead to dramatic changes in the child's condition, these occur only within the child-therapist relationship and do not carry over to the family context. The pattern of the child who "slips back" between treatments, e.g., stuttering, is common in behavioral disorders. We interpret "slippage" as homeostatic responses within a family aimed at restoring a previous equilibrium.

Individuals within a family organize their movements into behavior, and when this is integrated and coordinated with the behavior of another, an interaction is produced, e.g., a conversation or a fight. When people meet and interact regularly, they form a relationship, and its nature depends on the reinforcing qualities of the interactions on which it is based. The family is a set of such relationships, integrated to become compatible and interdependent within the system.

A mother and new baby develop a relationship by reinforcing each other's behavior so that it acquires communicative properties and, in so doing, establish a strong affectional bond. Within this and other similar family bonds, the child is led to further socialization, including the development of normal perceptual and social skills.

The aim of our treatment is to incorporate the child into a normal socializing affectional system. To do this, we attempt to set up a pattern of interactions within the family which will lead to affectional relationship with emphasis on socialization. The tools we use are those based on ordinary learning theory, behavior modification aimed not at individuals, but at relationships as the units of treatment.

Treatment

The three main phases of treatment are: preparation of the family; intensive treatment of the mother and child; and extended education of the child at a day center. All phases are under the direction of one specialist with assistants, and the whole family is always involved.

Preparation of the Family

After diagnostic assessment, the parents are told about our concepts of autism. They are then given a detailed preview of the treatment as follows (Clancy and McBride[5]):

1. The treatment will involve each family member in a program of activities over an extended period. Some idea is given of the general form of these activities and the reason for family participation.

2. The mother's special role is described, as are the stresses associated with the intensive treatment. Emphasis is placed on the temptation to abandon treatment when the child appears to be starving. Films of the details of procedures are shown.

3. The parents meet and learn the roles of each member of the therapeutic team. These are the director of treatment, the social worker who will coordinate the different aspects of each phase of treatment, and the therapists in the day center which the family visit.

The committment of the parents to the treatment is essential. Much can be achieved by gathering a number of families at a holiday camp. This usually proves to be the family's first enjoyable excursion with their child, among understanding neighbors. The holiday program includes an activity program for all members of the family, with group discussions among parents on the autistic process and its treatment. Parents are encouraged to experiment with changes in their responses to the child, with each family reinforcing the resolution of the others (Clancy[5]).

Intensive Treatment

We base intensive treatment on the correlation of feeding problems (Clancy et al.[4]) since the feeding situation provides a powerful context for intrusion on the child and for the promotion of affiliative interactions with the mother. The three requirements for intensive treatment are freedom of the mother from normal duties so that her attention is directed to the child at all times, an environment unfamiliar to the child, and continuous supervision of the mother and child. Hospitalization and medical supervision are necessary if the child is starving, though perhaps an apartment attached to the day care center would be adequate in other cases.

Procedure. On admission, the child is examined medically, and the mother is again given a detailed account of the forthcoming procedures. Abnormal objects to which the child was attached have been left at home, and these will now be denied him.

The next day, no breakfast is given, and the therapist offers the child an unfamiliar semisolid food mixed with his preferred food, made by his mother under supervision. To remove the social stress from the feeding the therapist sits beside, not opposite, the child and repeatedly offers the spoon, withdrawing it upon protest and reapproaching when the child becomes quiet. The child invariably refuses the food; the session lasts about 15 minutes and is then terminated without fuss. A similar meal is offered at successive mealtimes until the child begins to eat. Only water and nonnourishing drinks are given between meals. Breakfast need not be offered during the starvation period, but the therapist offers each other meal, seven days weekly. After each unsuccessful meal the mother is reassured and is encouraged to comfort the child. Her presence at meals is actively encouraged if she is helpful to the child, but she is given a choice. At all times she is free to move about the hospital, and she may go shopping or attend the day center with an active child. The mother must always remain with the child, engaging his interest when possible, distracting him from abnormal behaviors, and ignoring his tantrums, though naturally demands which provoke these should be reasonable. Giving preferred food is forbidden, but some mothers try. She should offer comfort, cuddles, and crooning to her lethargic child, who eventually passively accepts and later actively seeks comfort.

At this point the mother becomes anxious, aggressive, and uncertain in her relationship with the therapist, but protective and sympathetic to the child. Although this is a stressful period for all, its value is that child and mother are forced together into a comfort-giving and comfort-seeking relationship, which is strongly affiliative. All members of the team, especially the doctor, should support and reassure the mother.

Acceptance of food, from the second to the twelfth day, is immediately associated with enthusiastic social responses from therapist and mother, smiling, direct facial contact by gentle stroking of the cheek, and simple rewarding phrases. The mother should be demonstrative. With each successive meal the normal food is increased in amount and variety until the child is on a normal diet.

Mealtime as Playtime. As the therapist is present at meals, these become major teaching sessions. The day after eating starts, a playtime is begun, either before or after the meal. The aim is to introduce a range of social games and to develop a variety of social reward situations, along with simple perceptual skill training. Playtime continues throughout the intensive treatment, providing a basis for most mother-child activities. The range of demands can be illustrated through the activity of bubble blowing, which is the most attractive activity to autistic children. At first the mother blows bubbles at random until the child is sufficiently attentive for a demand to be made. Bubbles are then withheld until the child makes some positive indication, however slight, that he wants more, when his communication is immediately rewarded. More positive overtures are then required; for example, the child must take the mother's hand. These demands are achieved simply by waiting; the child may fuss, but apparently cannot resist the bubbles. The child must make eye contact on request, by looking up at the blower held at the mother's eye level. A specific or appropriate word like "mum" is next demanded. Words give way to simple and then complex sentences. This scale of demands is applied to all activities.

The mother resumes feeding when the child has taken one full meal enthusiastically, usually three or four after beginning to eat. Now he is eating voraciously, and it takes about two or three weeks to adjust to a normal level of intake; thereafter he eats a normal diet with normal preferences. The pair recommence regular attendance at the day center and are now included in all aspects of the program.

Further Behavioral Demands. The therapist now introduces new demands, handing each over to the mother. Eye contact, and later words and language, are demanded for each spoonful. The therapist bears the brunt of the child's anger, but when successful, quickly hands over to the watching mother who can be associated with the rewarding experience. But all participation is now on the mother's terms, in contrast to the past when all demands have been on the child's terms. Tantrums are now ineffective.

To gain eye contact, the therapist directs attention to the mother's face by holding the spoon at eye level. Language demands require cooperation; one makes the demand, and the mother prompts the response and rewards it promptly.

Self-Care Training. At the appropriate times simple training is given in dressing, bathing, and toileting. The mother is at first inept at this training and must be shown how to make the child successful at each step of these operations and then reward him with enthusiastic responses. Toilet training is achieved by administering an intestinal evacuant in decreasing doses. Successful responses are reinforced by praise, and the child is shown how the excrement is disposed of in the toilet. This program later continues at home where father is involved. The child is not allowed to wear diapers, and wet pants are not changed immediately. About one or two months are required for toilet training, and no strong pressures are imposed on the child.

The father, and if possible the siblings, join the child's meal-and playtimes when they visit the hospital and are encouraged to devise their own excursions, including eating in a public snack bar. Discussions continue daily with the mother, and less often with the father. Considerable time is given to normal development and child-rearing practices, and parents are encouraged to read in this area rather than about autism. The mother keeps her own diary of the intensive treatment, and this is maintained throughout.

Return Home. Where possible, the mother and child should spend one full weekend at home, with a well-defined program of activities for each member of the family with the child. These activities must be of a type already satisfying to the person concerned, and in the context of normal daily home life. The program must therefore be drawn up in consultation with the family. The child is not allowed solitude, and none of the previous abnormal habits are permitted. Certain rearrangements of the house may be necessary before the child returns; for example, objects previously collected and used abnormally must be destroyed and not replaced. It must be made clear to the family that misguided sympathy for the child only leads to the reestablishment of old patterns. Always the child must accede to the family's wishes, and not vice versa. Later there is room for permissiveness.

When the child has been eating a full normal diet for about a week, discharge is arranged for a weekend, so that the child is restored to full family life immediately. Without full preparation, there is likely to be slippage. The family must continue in a designated program of interactions which involve the child separately with each person at suitable times and in interactions which involve the family as a whole.

Education Program

The main purpose is to develop increasingly complex perceptual, language, and social skills under the guidance of specialists at the day center. The mother attends daily with the child for the first two to three weeks, and thereafter one day weekly. Regularly, perhaps once a term or semester, she attends full time for one to two weeks. The program is organized as follows:

1. Group sessions of four children, a therapist, and an assistant aim specifically to promote peer interaction and language as communication. Group excursions into the community occur daily, e.g., visiting shops and riding on public transportation. Each child also attends a normal preschool kindergarten with his mother, initially one day per week. As untrained assistants we employ high-grade mentally deficient young women, who cannot compete on the open labor market.
2. Individual training sessions are given to each child two or three times weekly separately in perceptual skills and language development (Brereton and Sattler[1]). Proficient skills are used as reinforcing activities for the training of weaker skills.

Language demands on the child increase gently as he becomes more socialized, and his own spontaneous efforts are built on to establish appropriate language use. Particular attention is given to developing concepts with their associated words. Colorful imaginative thought and its verbal expression are reinforced. Similarly, any latent sense of humor is fostered by teaching the child how to joke and be joked with. All language training is directed by a speech therapist.

The home program is reviewed regularly, at least monthly, with the family, either in a visit to the home by the therapist and the social worker or at the center. These visits are built around the diary maintained by the parents. The social worker's chief function, through discussion, is to reinforce efforts being made to improve the quality and variety of family interactive behavior. Where possible, the father attends the center and participates.

Initially the child's idiosyncratic behavior is discouraged. His activity is constantly directed, allowing limited opportunities for self-stimulating or cutoff behavior. With increasing socialization, the child's particular personal qualities become apparent. Now the directiveness in the treatment can be relaxed.

Contact with normal children at kindergarten increases until the child finally attends full time, visiting the center only for individual treatment sessions.

The ultimate aim of treatment is realistic schooling. Our criterion for discharge from the center if that the child's educational needs can now be met better by other appropriate agencies.

Assessment of Response

Sound-movie records made at regular intervals provide the best assessment of behavior change. At diagnosis, a full psychological assessment is attempted. This is repeated after the intensive treatment, thereafter at six-month intervals for one year, and then annually. Nonverbal tests such as the Merrill-Palmer are preferred, and the Illinois Test of Psycho-Linguistic Abilities is used diagnostically in relation to language. The Progressive Assessment Scale (Gunzberg) is useful for showing parents what progress is made in socialization abilities, and for encouraging them in their efforts.

Results

To date all intensive treatments (15) have been successful. Once commenced, the procedure should be continued until the child responds; otherwise his ability to resist social intrusion may be strengthened.

REFERENCES

1. Brereton, Le Guay B., and Sattler, J.: Cerebral Palsy: Basic Abilities. New South Wales, Australia, Mossman Spastic Centre, 1967.
2. Clancy, H.: The Autistic Playschool—An Evaluation. In: Curtis, J. (Ed.), An Autistic Playschool. Proceedings of a Family Holiday Venture. Mansfield, Victoria, Curtis, 1969.
3. Clancy, H., Dugdale, A., and Rendle-Short, J.: The Diagnosis of Infantile Autism. Develop. Med. Child Neurol. 11:432-442, 1969.
4. Clancy, H., Entch, M., and Rendle-Short, J.: Infantile Autism: The Correction of Feeding Abnormalities. Develop. Med. Child Neurol. 11:569-578, 1969.
5. Clancy, H., and McBride, G.: The Autistic Process and Its Treatment. J. Child Psychol. Psychiat. 10:233-244, 1970.
6. Clancy, H., and McBride, G.: The Isolation Syndrome. J. Child Psychol. Psychiat. (in press) 1971.

Comprehensive Residential Treatment of Adolescents

by Julian I. Barish, M.D., and William A. Schonfeld, M.D.

The admission of youthful patients to psychiatric hospitals, which began experimentally in the 1950s, has reached major proportions, with patients from 12 to 25 years of age comprising 50 to 80 per cent of psychiatric hospital populations. During these 20 years there has been a corresponding proliferation of hospital facilities for adolescents.[1] The time-honored term "residential treatment," formerly reserved for a few special programs, is now applied ambiguously to a variety of treatment facilities. A current definition of the nature and use of extended residential treatment for adolescents in hospitals seems indicated.

There are residential adolescent treatment centers other than those in hospitals; these have, basically, a social work or educational orientation. Social work settings, the oldest historically, emphasize group living, but also provide schooling and often psychotherapy, perhaps with psychological or psychiatric consultation. On the educational level, some special treatment schools and camps have a major focus on reeducation, both in academics and in social relationships. These facilities, too, may consult with other disciplines and may utilize concurrent psychotherapy. In contrast, the philosophy in hospitals blends the dynamic orientation of psychiatry with the biological orientation of clinical medicine. Hospitals may or may not provide schooling or programs dictated by the special needs of adolescents. If generalizations may be made, the first two forms of residential care emphasize the mobilization of healthy aspects of personality, whereas psychiatric hospitals have tended to stress the relief of psychopathology.

Unfortunately, there has been no formal evaluation of the relative effectiveness of the social, educational, and psychiatric approaches to residential treatment. However, a wholesome balance and a complete program would appear optimal. In recent years, a few psychiatric units have been developing more and more in that direction. A new type of hospital service is emerging for which the term "comprehensive residential treatment of adolescents" is suggested.

Editor's Note: The editor joins with the many friends of the late Dr. Schonfeld in mourning his recent death.

Definition

Comprehensive residential treatment implies, first, that an institution provides a complete milieu—one that meets the social, educational, and other growth and health needs of its adolescent patients; secondly, it implies a particular kind of long-term treatment in residence—an organized therapeutic use of the milieu and an integration of milieu therapy with other treatment modalities into a unified approach toward definitive therapeutic goals. Finally, if it is to be designated comprehensive, a residential treatment service must pay full attention to aftercare, arranging follow-up treatment, supportive services, and a smooth transition of the patient back to the community.

In short, comprehensive residential treatment is more than the management and treatment of adolescents away from home. The designation is not appropriate for facilities that limit themselves to crisis intervention, short-term hospitalization, or partial hospitalization; nor does it apply to day schools, halfway houses, group residences, or foster family placements, although there is admittedly some overlap in facilities and functions and many of these services are, by definition, included.

Basic Elements

Allowing for local variations in emphasis and style, there are basic elements that comprehensive residential treatment centers ideally hold in common.

Most psychiatric residential treatment centers for adolescents have a psychodynamic frame of reference, with extensions to include family and group dynamics. Psychodynamics, defined as the study of goal-directed behavior and its motivational forces, is derived from psychoanalysis, psychiatry, and psychology. It offers concepts of personality development, of motivating forces, and of mechanisms by which environmental forces are internalized. Psychodynamics has limitations in accommodating data on biological and on sociological levels, and other theoretical approaches such as general systems theory are being added. Psychodynamics, however, remains the most useful frame of reference available for the purpose.

In a psychodynamic frame of reference, problems are seen in terms of motivation as well as behavior and are viewed longitudinally as a function of personality development. Consequently, therapeutic goals involve more than relief of symptoms or change of maladaptive behavior; when possible, they aim at modification of basic motivation and at personality reconstruction; always, they are concerned with fostering healthy growth and development. Since achieving definitive goals requires considerable time, a typical treatment program will involve six months to several years in hospital and a like period of subsequent outpatient treatment.

Patients

Most adolescents in residential treatment are diagnosed as schizophrenia, personality disorders, or borderline states. These diagnoses do not fully convey the diversity of clinical problems, but they do imply long-standing ego defects, severe motivational conflicts, and pervasive disturbances of functioning. The usual problems of adolescence, often tumultuous in themselves, are intensified and distorted. The customary themes and conflicts about impulse control, body image, dependency versus independence, peer relationships, sexual adequacy, identity, competition, authority, etc., are presented. Also appearing in magnified form is the adolescent propensity for acting out—repetitive, symbolic, behavioral communication of anxieties and conflicts, at times in self-destructive and socially disturbing forms, which present both real dangers and unique opportunities for meaningful therapeutic intervention.

The number of adolescents makes a substantial difference in the character of a hospital milieu. A few adolescents may dominate a mixed adolescent-adult service, but without providing the minimum number necessary to make practical the required special staff and program. Moreover, the interactions in a sizable peer group are essential for residential treatment. Too large a number, however, makes management difficult. Units of 10 to 20 adolescents offer a suitable balance.

Hospitals must be selective in the numbers and types of patients they treat. A single facility may not be able to deal with the full range of adolescent problems. The use of drugs, so prevalent in our adolescent subculture, is not managed easily, and some hospitals avoid drug problems. Other hospitals set an arbitrary age limit for acceptance; this should not supplant biological and social development as determining criteria. A serious deficiency in some states has been the exclusion of youths over 16 years from adolescent programs, not as a result of psychiatric judgment, but because education is not compulsory after 16.

Staff

Because of their energy, rebelliousness, and varied needs, adolescents require greater numbers of supervising personnel and a wider range of professional disciplines than do other age groups. More important than numbers, however, are the qualifications of professional staff, since therapeutic use of self is a *sine qua non* for all personnel in comprehensive residential treatment. The first qualification is the possession of certain difficult-to-define personality traits. One such trait is tolerance for adolescents—who do have a knack of threatening defenses and of evoking anxiety. Adolescents themselves say that attributes such as flexibility, firmness, sincerity, fairness, self-confidence, a desire to be of help, and the like are desirable.

Beyond personality traits, the paramedical professional staff require expertise derived from training and, especially, experience. Key hospital personnel should be assigned to work with adolescents as their sole responsibility so that they may regard adolescents as a major professional interest. Some professionals see adolescents merely as troublemakers, which they often are; but an experienced and sensitive person will ask, "Why?" and will react to the trouble appropriately. The psychiatrists who work with adolescents should also have special training and experience with this age group. (It is, in fact, important that all general psychiatric residents, as well as residents in child psychiatry, have supervised treatment of adolescents as part of their training. In addition, more opportunities for advanced training in adolescent psychiatry are needed to qualify psychiatrists as directors of adolescent services.

Therapeutic Modalities

A comprehensive residential treatment milieu has immediately available a wide range of treatment modalities that can be integrated into individually planned programs. These include milieu therapy, individual psychotherapy, group therapy and family therapy, psychopharmacotherapy, and the organic therapies, plus the so-called ancillary therapies: educational, occupational recreational, art, and perhaps music and dance therapy; as well as counseling in family relationships, in legal matters, in social skills, and in educational and vocational placements. Obviously, the choice and manner of application of these modalities varies considerably.

Milieu therapy, a vague entity, is not a specific treatment modality, but is nonetheless a potent therapeutic force. It comprises all the basic elements of milieu described herein and serves as a vehicle for the other modalities of treatment, but it is more than the sum total of these. It requires a coherent social organization that provides an extensive treatment context and which coordinates and integrates the various treatment modalities. According to Abroms, the aim of milieu therapy is to direct social contacts and treatment experience synergistically toward specific, realistic therapeutic goals.[2]

Whereas milieu therapy serves as a context and an integrating force for the therapeutic process, the core modality of treatment is individual psychotherapy, adapted by the therapist in his own style to each patient's needs. If milieu therapy is the vehicle of the treatment process, ongoing psychotherapy is its steering mechanism. Comprehensive residential treatment begins with a diagnostic evaluation in which a psychiatric case study is supplemented by the daily observations of professional staff. The therapist becomes the leader of a treatment team composed of representatives of various professional disciplines who interact with, and try to understand, the patients and each other. Individual psychotherapy provides an irreplaceable means of understanding a patient's unfolding dynamic pattern; further, the emotional context of the one-to-one relationship offers therapeutic leverage that is different from that of other modalities; finally, it serves as a check and balance for the otherwise group-oriented residential treatment.

Group therapy is also important in that it provides a controlled dynamic interaction and confrontation with peers. Psychopharmacotherapy is useful in relieving certain target symptoms such as excessive anxiety, depression, or decompensation so as to facilitate psychotherapy, education, and socialization.

Structure

"Structure," in psychiatric jargon, refers to a regulated style of daily living. Patients are required to arise and retire on schedule, to eat meals at regular times, to attend activities and keep treatment appointments, to dress within prescribed modes, to observe telephone and visiting restrictions, to avoid behavior designated as objectionable and to follow other local grounds rules.

Each of these facets of living has its own set of psychodynamic meanings. Morning awakening, for example, can become a repetitive problem in which fear of failure, defensive anger, depression, and hopelessness are expressed. Similarly, going to bed at night elicits fears of helplessness and loss of control. The management of each requires skill and patience. However, these focal points of arising and retiring can also be the occasions of the most significant communication between patients and staff.

Structure helps recompensate a disorganized adolescent, sets limits for one who acts out, and gives all youth the symbols of authority to interact with. It provides the behavior control advocated by Hendrickson and Holmes as essential for residential treatment of adolescents.[3] Structure and behavior control are necessary components of dynamic residential therapy; they should not, however, be so rigid as to prevent spontaneity or, indeed, all acting out. To reiterate, adolescent acting out often provides valuable opportunities for therapeutic intervention, through psychotherapeutic sanctions, peer disapproval, and, hopefully, insight as to motivation.

Activities

Whereas the scheduling of activities is an integral part of the structure of a hospital, and the need for a schedule is similar for adults, the type and variety of activities are different in an adolescent program.

Schooling is the customary occupation of adolescents and is appropriately the key activity in their residential programs. In some settings, the school is an integral part of the institution. It may be modeled after a community school, or it may operate along the lines of educational therapy. Individual tutoring and a flexible curriculum are needed in order to meet the requirements and adjust to the limitations of certain patients. It is important to offer high school credit for courses completed. In other institutions, adolescent patients attend the local junior or senior high school or are enrolled in neighboring tutoring schools. In still others, correspondence courses are utilized. Several universities with hospital programs for college students use their own academic facilities. Douady et al.[4] report that a network of special hospitals for college students in France have the prerequisite of continuation of studies by each patient during treatment.

A variety of additional activities (physical, mechanical, artistic) are required to match the wide range of adolescent interests and are integrated into the therapeutic program. Nontherapeutic activities, too, are necessary to allow a respite from concentrated treatment. Youths also need a time and a place to which they may go off by themselves to read, think, or cry. Activities within the surrounding community also help to minimize the cloistered effect of residential treatment and ease transition back after discharge. Further, activities oriented to helping others serve as a counterforce to self-preoccupation and to the fascination with drug-induced perceptual experiences so currently common among adolescents.

Housing

There has been much debate, without reaching a definite conclusion, about adolescents in hospitals having separate quarters or sharing them with adults. There are advantages to each arrangement. With separate housing, a peer culture is established, more adolescents are amenable to treatment, and there is greater therapeutic leverage. With shared housing, particularly when adults greatly outnumber the adolescents, acting out is less and behavior control is easier. Ideally, both arrangements should be available, since some youths respond better to one than to the other. Realistically, the choice usually depends on local conditions such as the availability of space and staff. Separate housing is of less consequence than separate programs and a well-trained multidisciplinary staff under the supervision of a psychiatrist specializing in adolescents' problems.

Families

The patient's family may not be living on the hospital grounds, but it is nonetheless a vital element of the hospital milieu. An effective system of communicating with parents is essential, since they can reinforce or undermine therapeutic efforts, depending on their own needs and on how well they are coordinated with the treatment. As a minimum standard for parents' involvement, they should be kept informed about the patient's status and progress, and should have counseling to improve their understanding of the patient and their dealings with him. In many cases, of course, more elaborate treatment for families is indicated.

Group Dynamics

Conscious use of informal and planned interactions is an essential ingredient of a residential treatment program. Group dynamics may be defined simply as the interaction of individuals with each other and with social institutions, but under this rubric are found the most complex and least understood therapeutic phenomena. As Redl has indicated, we do not have adequate concepts, or even the language, to describe fully the multiple, subtle transactions among people in a hospital.[5] Yet, these transactions exert a powerful influence, both positive and negative, on the treatment process.

Aftercare

Abrupt discharge or faulty aftercare without adequate supportive and rehabilitative services can undermine an otherwise positive result of residential treatment. For gradual transition back into the community, a comprehensive service may be required to arrange continued treatment, educational or vocational counseling, school or job placement, housing or surrogate family, and social contacts. The range of services may be supplied by the institution itself or through cooperation with other agencies in the community. Perhaps, for most efficient operation, comprehensive residential centers should be part of a broad continuum of facilities so organized as to permit close cooperation and ease of transfer. This may be made possible by the community mental health program.

Indications for Comprehensive Residential Treatment

Few authors mention specific indications for long-term residential treatment. Beckett notes that adolescents are usually referred for inpatient treatment because of behavior that "adult society considers boisterous, aggressive or violent." [6] But use of that criterion alone would qualify most teenagers for residential treatment at some time during their development. Easson cites two basic criteria for residential treatment of an adolescent—a deficit in ego strength manifested by an inability to control drives and impulses, *and* a lack of emotional capability to form meaningful relationships.[7]

There are other factors to consider. The prescription of comprehensive residential treatment should be made only after a thorough evaluation of the patient, his family, and his social environment gives positive indication that it is the treatment of choice. Furthermore, the recommendation should be carried out only if there is a hospital available which can treat him effectively. Each factor and the whole configuration must be considered. Is the adolescent's problem pervasive and severe enough to warrant such intensive and extensive treatment, and will it be amenable to a comprehensive residential approach? Is he maladjusted in multiple areas—family, school, social, and sexual? Is the family interaction pathogenic and does it perpetuate the problem? Are there significant positive forces in school or in peer relationships which should be preserved? Can the adolescent and his family be helped to use the hospital experience constructively? Which of the hospitals under consideration are likely to manage the patient and his family most effectively? How long a period of treatment is needed? Is it financially feasible for the family? These are representative questions that a referring person or an admitting psychiatrist must ask himself. Aftercare planning should also begin at this stage. Can the patient return to his family after discharge from the hospital? What other arrangements will be necessary for aftercare?

Adolescents are at a particularly malleable stage of development. Comprehensive residential treatment, therefore, is a powerful therapeutic force, since it supplies a maximum of external support, direction, and influence. When carefully designed and properly used, such programs can effectively treat some problem adolescents who cannot be helped in any other way—and may be life-saving.

Conversely, comprehensive residential treatment can also be a destructive force. Easson cautions that injudicious or ill-timed use of inpatient therapy may not only fail to benefit the patient but may also produce emotional regression and personality stunting.[7] Unnecessary or badly planned hospital placement may handicap an adolescent emotionally and intellectually. Consequently, the prescription of comprehensive residential treatment must be made with great care. Less radical methods of treatment are to be considered first, keeping in mind, however, that procrastination in prescribing residential treatment when it is the method of choice may lose valuable time and may conceivably permit preventable tragedies. In short, fine clinical judgment is required. When in doubt, a trial period in a comprehensive facility may clarify whether extended treatment is indicated.

Comprehensive residential treatment may follow crisis-oriented therapy, but the indications for the two are quite different. Dangerous behavior or exposure to excessive stress may be sufficient indication for short-term psychiatric hospitalization, but not for continued residential treatment. A youth who is a drug abuser or even a potential suicide is not necessarily a candidate for comprehensive residential treatment. Nor should hospitals be used as tools of popular prejudice to remove from society those youths who do not accept conventional concepts. Only those adolescents who show positive indications for, and who can benefit from, the experience should be considered.

The choice of a hospital is crucial. To judge whether an institution can be expected to treat a specific patient effectively, the prescriber should know the strengths and limitations of the institution's particular milieu, its treatment philosophy and practice, and its attitude toward aftercare. A poorly matched patient and residential service may result in a treatment failure or in equally undesirable custodial care.

By definition, comprehensive residential treatment should be part of a total treatment program for the adolescent and his family. For that reason its prescription is best made by a professional who not only can make a suitable evaluation, but also, if possible, maintain contact with the hospital, the family, and the patient. He may be of immeasurable help in minimizing the anxieties and guilt inevitably evoked by the recommendation of psychiatric hospitalization, in overcoming family resistances as they arise during the course of treatment, and in ensuring continuity of care after discharge.

The prescriber of comprehensive treatment can give no positive prognostication or definite promise about its outcome. With such a new, potent, and complex tool, uncertain results are not surprising. Hopefully, as methods employed are developed further, their positive indications and inherent limitations will be more precisely defined.

REFERENCES

1. Hartmann, E., Glasser, B. A., Greenblatt, M., Solomon, M. H., and Levinson, D. J.: Psychiatric Inpatient Treatment of Adolescents: A Review of Clinical Experience, Chapter I. In: Adolescents in a Mental Hospital. New York, Grune & Stratton, Inc., 1968.
2. Abroms, G. M.: Defining Milieu Therapy. Arch. Gen. Psychiat. (Chicago) 21:553-560, 1969.
3. Hendrickson, W. J., and Holmes, D. J.: Control of Behavior as a Crucial Factor in Intensive Psychiatric Treatment in an All Adolescent Ward. Amer. J. Psychiat. 115:969, 1959.
4. Douady, D., Jeanguyot, M.-Th., Neel, D., Danon-Boileau, H., Lab, P., Brousselle, A., and Levy, E.: L'Organisation des Cliniques Medico-Psychologiques de la Fondation Sante des Etudiants de France. Rev. Neuropsychiat. Infant 15:505-535, 1967.
5. Redl, F.: Aggression in Adolescence. Society for Adolescent Psychiatry, Annual Lecture, New York, Oct. 26, 1967. (Unpublished.)
6. Beckett, P. G. S.: Adolescents Out of Step: Their Treatment in a Psychiatric Hospital. Detroit, Wayne University Press, 1965.
7. Easson, W. M.: The Severely Disturbed Adolescent. New York, International Universities Press, 1969.

PART II

ADULT PSYCHOTHERAPEUTIC TECHNIQUES

The Problem of Buridan's Ass: Psychotherapy for Choice

by Z. J. Lipowski, M.D.

This is not an excursion into animal psychiatry. It is an attempt to formulate some implications for mental health and psychotherapy of a major change in our social environment: The key issues to be discussed concern affluence, attractive stimulus surfeit, and the related conflicts of choice. The parable of Buridan's ass, which could not choose which of two sacks of oats to approach and died of starvation, is a fitting analogy for some dilemmas of contemporary man.[1] This classical example of an approach-approach type of conflict should not, of course, be taken literally: a fatal outcome is not usually at stake. There is, however, convincing experimental evidence that an unresolved conflict involving equally attractive alternatives may lead to neurotic behavior.[2] What concerns us here are some manifestations of the "malaise of affluence"[3] and their relevance for the mental health professions.

Formulation of the Problem

In two recent articles[1,4] this writer has put forth a set of propositions which he called a theory of attractive stimulus overload or surfeit theory. It is germane to recapitulate these postulates as a basis for discussion.

It is an inherent characteristic of the affluent, postindustrial society that it subjects its members to an overload of attractive stimuli (or information inputs). "Attractive" in this context refers to those external stimuli capable of arousing appetitive and approach responses in individuals on whom they impinge. "Overload" connotes a subject's relative inability to choose among and/or approach equally (for him) desirable goals. There are thus two necessary

18

conditions for the overload: a social environment providing an overabundance of attractive stimuli of a high level of diversity, appeal, and frequency; and a population of individuals responding to and having difficulties with the information input. It is proposed that these conditions are widely prevalent in affluent societies which provide tempting options, both material and symbolic, on a scale unprecedented in man's history. There are not only a vast quantity and variety as well as easy availability of objects to possess and consummate, but also a whole range of symbolic values and goals to choose from and pursue. The latter include diverse work and leisure opportunities, styles of living, and modes of social and sexual interaction. In addition, there is the influential ethos of the "psychology of more." [5] Our consumer-oriented economy, advertising, and the messages of the mass media combine to promote an ever-growing number and diversity of wants and expectations. And here creeps in the malaise observed by students of behavioral economics: "The more we feel we must have, the smaller the chance of gratifying all our wants and the greater the possibility of great expectations making for stress, tension, and anxiety." [3]

The overabundance of attractive goals to strive for has serious, psychological consequences. There is an analogy here to the stressful effects of both overload and deprivation of sensory inputs. One may regard attractive stimulus overload as a special category of the general information overload which is one of the pervasive features of a technological society. This category is distinguished by its *meaning,* one which evokes in many subjects appetitive arousal and related approach-action tendencies. Attractive information inputs have different effects depending on the economic condition of various individuals. The economically underprivileged who respond to such inputs have a restricted freedom of choice and consummation. "The poor feel discriminated against and alienated; . . . they demand and press for immediate change in their situation." [3] The well-to-do face a different dilemma: one of choice. Yet psychological and temporal limitations restrict their ability to approach and consummate. There is thus ample opportunity for approach-approach variety of intrapsychic conflict, epitomized by the parable of Buridan's ass. This form of conflict is not new to man, but its frequency and intensity in the affluent societies are a novel feature. This conclusion seems obvious and yet its psychological implications have not sufficiently influenced psychodynamic theory. The latter has been built around the conception of the approach-avoidance type of conflict as one possessing a powerful pathogenic potential. Anxiety, guilt, defense mechanisms, and resultant neuroses are all predicated on an intrapsychic conflict between unacceptable approach tendencies and the opposing avoidance forces. These theoretical constructs are still valid and clinically useful, but need to be supplemented.

In contrast, the conflict occasioned by attractive but incompatible options has been traditionally regarded as easily solved.[1] This assumption must be revised to take into account compelling realities of our contemporary existence which call for a broadening of our concepts of intrapsychic conflict and revision of its role in eliciting psychopathology. Rangell[6] agrees that "to the traditional meaning of psychoanalytic conflict as an opposition between forces . . . is added a second meaning of conflict as a 'choice,' a 'decision dilemma' . . . a crucial type of intrasystemic conflict within the ego."

Coping with Attractive Stimulus Overload

The particular strategies and effectiveness of coping with approach-approach-derived stresses will be influenced by factors within the individual and his social environment.[4] The generation brought up in the postwar affluence, social change, and spectacular development of the mass media, particularly television, has been especially exposed to a high degree of attractive stimulation from early life on. Many parents have had their own unresolved difficulties with the same problems, have offered inadequate models and guidelines for choice, and have implicitly or explicitly questioned and defied former value systems and norms of behavior. This further complicates the sharply contrasting world views confronting the young: on the one hand, immense possibilities for gratification; on the other, violence, vicious competition, and the prospect of global annihilation. This promotes a sense of urgency to choose and consummate, but offers no credible values on which to base decision making. Youths, particularly at the college level, may then resort to several strategies:

1. *Selective Responsivity.* This may be a partly innate, partly learned capacity to respond with appetitive arousal and to choose only a manageable proportion of available options. This is an adaptive strategy which, as noted by Halleck,[7] challenges parents and educators and the solution for which has largely eluded them.

2. *Avoidance of Excess Stimuli and Related Conflicts.* This may take various forms: withdrawal; absorption in some activity, be it inner fantasy (aided by drugs or other stratagems) or outward directed pursuits.

3. *Active Stimulus Seeking and Repeated Attempts at Consummation.* Such ceaseless activity and striving are usually productive of short-lived satiety followed by more stimulus hunger and search. It appears that adherents of this strategy have a low threshold for appetitive arousal, respond impulsively, and are least capable of selective responsivity and enduring gratification.

4. *Avoidance of Commitment.* This strategy implies a protean existence[8] characterized by frequent tentative approaches to and sampling of many options without any firm choice and sustained consummation. This solution, despite its outward appearance of liveliness and richness, seems to be a frequent source of a sense of emptiness and futility so well described by Fairbairn in his discussion of schizoid individuals.[9]

5. *Suspended Action.* This implies a stalemate often accompanied by frustration, resentment, and apathy. It is the closest human analogy to Buridan's ass. Some individuals attempt to break out of the painful impasse by periodic outbursts of frantic activity, even violence, followed by return to the passive stance.

This tentative list of coping strategies with the dilemmas outlined here is not exhaustive. The strategies overlap and may be resorted to at different times by the same individual. The list is presented to underscore the potential undesirable effects of the attractive stimulus overload and approach-approach conflicts on the stability of individuals and society. It raises the question: what can psychiatrists do to help alleviate problems contributed by the "malaise of affluence"?

Implications for Clinical Psychiatry

The main purpose of the preceding discussion was to draw attention to what this writer perceives as a major psychological consequence of the current social change. It is relevant for the young and their parents, patients and their therapists. One may observe it most readily in the so-called borderline personalities in whom it may both play a part in the development of emotional instability and heighten the latter as a result of the usually impaired capacity for choice making.

The challenge to psychiatrists is twofold: prevention and alleviation. The former must involve methods of child rearing and education. Specifically, one would have to advise parents and educators how to protect children against stimulus overload and help them learn to choose and make decisions. Such advice cannot be given as yet for lack of relevant knowledge. More is known about the effects of stimulus deprivation and more emphasis is put on providing enriched environments for disadvantaged children than on coping with information overload. Thus prevention must await results of future research. All we can do at present is to draw attention to the problem as this writer and others before him have done.[2,10,11]

What can we offer those individuals who already experience serious difficulties in managing attractive stimulus overload and choice conflicts? Can traditional methods of psychotherapy achieve this specific goal? Some therapists seem to believe that successful resolution of "infantile" id-ego conflicts will automatically facilitate choosing and decision making. This assumption is an act of faith. It ignores the aspects of current social change discussed here which make such an outcome far from certain. Therapeutic approaches need to be modified to meet new adaptational challenges.

Techniques of Therapy

A hallmark of the proposed approach is the emphasis on *education for choice* and training in *decision making*. The relevant techniques are based on the following premises:

1. The higher the number of attractive options, the more difficult it is to decide and choose.
2. The more differentiated a person's hierarchy of values is, the easier the choice.
3. Subjective strength of values increases in response to rewards accruing from their pleasurable consummation.
4. Clear formulation of both attractive options and one's personal values facilitates choice behavior.
5. Major intrapersonal blocks to decision making include ambivalence and fear of making the wrong choice and thus risk possible irreparable loss of rejected alternative.
6. According to a principle of decision making, when selections among multiattribute alternatives are involved, individuals test "various frames of mind until they find one whose associated subjective weights give one alternative the clearest advantage over its competitors."[12] It is proposed that this process may be facilitated by psychotherapeutic intervention.

The techniques of psychotherapy to be described do not supersede those currently used but only supplement them. They follow logically from the above premises and include:

1. Clarification. Clarification involves cooperative effort by therapist and patient to bring into the latter's full awareness both the values and options attractive to him. The therapist plays an active role by formulating as clearly as possible all alternatives which the patient communicates explicitly or indirectly, as in the form of free associations and dream content.

2. Weighing of Alternatives. This technique involves repeated presentation by the therapist of the alternatives which have been formulated. The patient is encouraged to discuss the advantages and disadvantages of each alternative in the light of both his objectives and capacities as well as the realities of his current life situation. As a result of this interaction, the number of considered options is brought to a minimum and only those remain which are almost equal in attractiveness.

3. Resolution of Approach-Approach Conflicts. The preceding technique leads to an intensification of this type of conflict. It is a subjectively unpleasant state characterized by mounting anxiety, ambivalence, and vacillation. The therapist encourages the patient to imagine vividly that he has already decided which alternative to choose, and to talk about his feelings. The patient experiments in fantasy in a manner similar to a phobic patient who is asked to imagine himself exposed to the phobic object or situation. This is a preparation for action which is aided by the discomfort of being in a state of conflict and the wish to end it. The latter is resolved by arriving at a decision and acting on it.

The main impediments to conflict resolution are not only the attractive attributes of the alternatives but also their negative features which involve varying degrees of uncertainty and risk regarding the outcome of choice. Further, individuals differ with regard to the degree to which they are prone to experience ambivalence and tolerate uncertainty. Obsessional and impulsive subjects may be viewed as representing two opposite types of pathologic decision making. They both react to the probability of risk and the stress of choice conflict, but in contrasting manner: by ineffective ruminations and inaction, or by precipitate decision and headlong plunge into action, respectively. The techniques described here must be adjusted to the type of patient treated. With the obsessional patient one has to proceed as if he were morbidly fearful of choosing. This implies a form of "desensitization" method by repeated "trial" decisions and active encouragement to resolve the choice conflict by pointing out that certainty is unattainable and the stalemate probably more painful than the outcome of choice. With an impulsive patient one must often warn against the consequences of escape from conflict by a hasty and premature decision.

There is one other category of patients who present marked difficulties with decision making: those who fear commitment, not unlike the claustrophobic's dread of closed places. A corollary of this is a fear of double loss: of freedom of action and of the discarded choice. Patients of this type often have a weak sense of their own identity and undifferentiated personal value systems. They may feel overwhelmed by the wealth of options which they find attractive and sometimes attempt to cope with this overload by evolving a conviction that nothing attracts them strongly enough or at all. These patients should be helped in defining more sharply the hierarchy of their values and goals. They should be encouraged to experiment in action with one of their preferred options, as this may provide positive feedback in the form of pleasurable consummation which can in turn enhance their sense of competence and identity as well as their hierarchy of values.

4. *Dealing with Postdecision Blues.* Some patients experience a keen sense of loss and grief after making a substantial decision. This is particularly likely to happen in the case of commitment-shy individuals. Allowing the patient to express his mourning for the discarded alternative should be combined with an attempt to counteract idealization of what he gave up. Some individuals have a marked tendency to embellish what they lose or discard and to make a myth of it which overshadows anything they have chosen and possess. It is crucial for the therapist to identify this tendency, bring it to the patient's attention, and help him search for its developmental roots. The goal is to prevent formation of new myths and give up the already established ones. This therapeutic task is important as it involves removal of a major impediment to choice making in the future. This type of response to choice and commitment is contrasted with that in which the person makes up for the given-up alternative by enhancing the attractiveness of the chosen one and, perhaps, depreciating the discarded one. These two attitudes may represent enduring personality traits of interest to both decision theorists and clinicians.

This condensed account is unavoidably oversimplified. Like all such accounts, it is more formal and intellectual than its application in actual practice. The principles described are applicable to both individual and group therapy. Their ultimate aim is to help the patient build his own hierarchy of values which is the single most effective factor in any coping strategy with attractive information overload and related conflicts of choice. Thus the impasse of Buridan's ass may be avoided.

A brief clinical illustration may help flesh out the problem and technique: This 28-year-old married mother of one sought psychotherapy to help her solve decision dilemmas involving all major aspects of her life. Her husband had been transferred to another city but she postponed joining him and considered leaving him. She was attracted to her husband as a reliable man and the only one with whom she could have orgasm. At the same time she felt attracted to three other men, each of whom represented a different set of desirable features. She had affairs with all three and was unable to decide which of them had the most to offer her in the long run and in comparison to her husband. The patient had trained as a nurse and enjoyed her work, at which she was successful. At the same time she had a strong desire to be an actress and was taking drama classes which she enjoyed no less than nursing and was praised by experienced actors. She also wrote poetry. She expressed desire to be unattached to a man, to do what she pleased, free from commitments; at the same time, she talked about wanting the security and warmth of a stable relationship with one man and of her need for sustained effort and accomplishment in one area and a settled, committed life. She was unable to make decisions and choose from among the largely incompatible alternatives and felt frustrated by the stalemate itself to the point of considering suicide as a way out.

Therapy consisted of 14 twice-weekly sessions. It included all aspects of the method described above. At first the patient complained of depression, tension, and confusion about her identity and goals. In the early sessions a successful attempt was made to help her put into words the conflicting self-images and desires, available options, and the extent of their congruence with her needs and values. This clear formulation of alternatives to choose from was followed by lifting of depression and the pervasive feeling of being anguished and trapped. The phase of weighing of the alternatives followed and evoked an intense search of her past experiences, particularly with her parents, for clues about the origins of her clashing values and goals. This phase was accompanied by expressions of shifting transference and counter-transference toward the therapist, as he came to represent significant persons in her past. She complained bitterly about her easy responsivity to too many choices coming her way and her relative inability to give up any of them. She gradually discarded two of her lovers, and her alternatives were reduced to a choice between her husband and a married lover with whom she had had a passionate affair prior to therapy and whom she tended to idealize despite the fact that he refused to leave his wife for her. The other pair of alternatives involved nursing and devotion to others on the one hand, and artistic expression on the other. She contacted her former lover to test his response and also visited her husband to assess the likely consequences of saving the marriage. Throughout this phase the therapist confined herself to neutral interpretations and repeated presentation of the alternatives as she had formulated them. This represents clinical application and reinforcement of premise 6 (see above) based on decision theory. At first the patient resented his refusal to tell her what to do, but after a series of reappraisals she made her decision to join her husband, return to part-time nursing, and give up acting, which, she felt, compounded her confusion about her own identity. She decided to express herself artistically in writing poetry, which was less conflictual and more feasible. During this last stage of therapy there were a few stormy episodes when the patient decided to give up her lover not only as a potential mate but also as a yearned-for ideal that made her husband look dull by comparison. It was a grief reaction to the loss of a cherished daydream and ended in her acknowledging that the real man was not without serious flaws. Thus the mourning (the "postdecision blues") for the lost ideal and alternative was overtly expressed, abreacted, and worked through.

This brief example illustrates the results of application of the focal approach described above. It must be clear that the latter is not incompatible with the full use of the traditional techniques of free association, dream analysis, interpretation, clarification, and emotional support. Nor does it ignore the importance of approach-avoidance-type conflicts. Not all patients respond as readily and rapidly as this intelligent and highly motivated woman has done. The writer has used this method in both brief psychotherapy involving weeks and prolonged treatments extending over 2 to 4 years. He recommends it particularly for late adolescents and young adults presenting various constellations of impaired capacity for decision and choice whether chronic or brought to the fore by a life crisis. Lewin[13] was right when he wrote that approach-approach conflicts are relatively easy to solve unless "questions are involved which cut deeply into the life of the individual." Such questions are not new to man, but tend to affect more individuals than ever before as a result of current social changes.

REFERENCES

1. Lipowski, Z. J.: The Conflict of Buridan's Ass or Some Dilemmas of Affluence: The Theory of Attractive Stimulus Overload. Amer. J. Psychiat. 127–273-279, 1970.
2. Masserman, J. H.: The Effect of Positive-Choice Conflicts on Normal and Neurotic Monkeys. Amer. J. Psychiat. 120:481-484, 1963.
3. Katona, G., Strumpel, B., and Zahn, E.: Aspirations and Affluence. New York, McGraw-Hill Book Co., Inc., 1971.
4. Lipowski, Z. J.: Surfeit of Attractive Information Inputs: A Hallmark of Our Environment. Behav. Sci. 16:467-471, 1971.
5. Looft, W. R.: The Psychology of More. Amer. Psychol. 26:561-565, 1971.
6. Rangell, L.: Choice-Conflict and the Decision-Making Function of the Ego: A Psychoanalytic Contribution to Decision Theory. Int. J. Psychoanal. 50:599-602, 1969.
7. Halleck, S.: Therapy of the Alienated College Student. Curr. Psychiat. Ther. 10:76-82, 1970.
8. Lifton, R. J.: Protean Man. Arch. Gen. Psychiat. (Chicago) 24:298-304, 1971.

9. Fairbairn, W. R. D.: Psychoanalytic Studies of the personality. London, Tavistock
    Publications, 1952.
10. Miller, J. G.: Information Input Overload and Psychopathology. Amer. J. Psychiat.
    116:695-704, 1960.
11. Spitz, R. A.: The Derailment of Dialogue. J. Amer. Psychoanal. Ass. 12:752-775,
    1964.
12. Shepard, R. N.: On Subjectively Optimum Selections Among Multi-attribute Alterna-
    tives. In: Edwards, W., and Tversky, A., Decision Making. Baltimore, Penguin
    Books, 1967, pp. 267-283.
13. Lewin, K.: A Dynamic Theory of Personality. New York, McGraw-Hill Book Co., Inc.,
    1935.

Advances in Behavior Therapy

by Joseph Wolpe, M.D.

Since this is the first review of behavior therapy to appear in *Current Psychiatric Therapies,* it is necessary to define its scope. The unadaptive habits that make up the field of psychiatry are all the result of one or both of two classes of processes—physical pathology (mainly lesions of nerve cells or biochemical abnormalities) and learning. Unadaptive habits that have been acquired by learning may reasonably be expected to be eliminated by learning. Laboratory studies have given us a number of principles and paradigms of learning that have generated clinically usable methods. *Behavior therapy* (also known as *conditioning therapy*) is the widely accepted generic name for procedures for overcoming unadaptive learned habits by applying experimentally established principles. The commonest targets of behavior therapy have been neurotic habits (especially anxiety habits) and those habits of schizophrenics that are attributable to learning.

Two kinds of principles are commonly used. Operant (instrumental) conditioning principles are applied to motor and ideomotor habits, counter-conditioning principles to emotional habits. The essence of operant conditioning is to arrange for desired behavior to be followed by "reinforcement" (reward) and for undesired behavior not to be so followed. The effect of a skillfully arranged schedule is progressively to displace the undesired behavior by the desired.[1,2]

The paradigm most often applied to the treatment of unadaptive emotional habits (especially anxiety) was derived from observations on experimental neuroses. We define anxiety as the particular organism's characteristic pattern of autonomic responses to noxious stimulation. An experimental neurosis is essentially a very strong anxiety (fear) response habit conditioned in a laboratory animal by any of a variety of methods in which severe anxiety is elicited in the animal while it is confined in a small cage.[3-5] The habit is extremely persistent. The anxiety is at its strongest in the experimental cage, inhibiting eating even if the animal is starving. In 1948, having made cats neurotic by a method approximating that of Masserman, I found, as had Masserman,[15] that they could be "cured." The method I used was feeding in a place remotely similar to the experimental situation until anxiety declined to zero there, and then in progressively more similar situations.[6,7] Apparently, feeding reciprocally inhibited anxiety and, in consequence, produced decondi-

27

tioning of the anxiety habit. The practical conclusion to which this led was that any response that could inhibit neurotic anxiety might be usable as a deconditioning agent.

In clinical practice the most widely adopted anxiety-inhibiting agent has been deep muscle relaxation,[8] and most often in the content of systematic desensitization,[7,9] a technique in which the relaxed patient is directed to *imagine* anxiety-evoking situations in "hierarchical" order (i.e., of increasing strength)—each of them repeated until it ceases to evoke anxiety before the next stronger image is introduced. Other common anxiety-inhibiting agents are assertive responses, sexual responses, and the emotional responses of the patient to the therapist. The last is "transference" in the loose sense. Such responses, when other than anxiety, apparently inhibit anxiety elicited by verbal stimuli during interviews, bringing about a good deal of inadvertent benefit in all interview therapies. The same kind of beneficial effects occur with systematically introduced anxiety-evoking stimuli.

The deconditioning of anxiety has a preeminent place in the treatment of neurosis because behavior analysis—the investigation of stimulus-response relations that must always precede behavior therapy—has shown anxiety to lie at the core of almost all neuroses, excepting classical hysteria. Thus psychosomatic states, obsessions and compulsions, character neuroses, sexual inadequacies, stuttering, and most other neuroses respond to deconditioning the anxiety habits to which these various manifestations are secondary.[10]

Research in behavior therapy has been increasing rapidly, especially in the past decade. Krasner,[11] in preparing an extensive review, compiled a bibliography of over 4000 items. The present review will be confined, in the main, to research of practical import.

Systematic Desensitization

We shall first consider advances related to this technique because of its relevance to the commonest cases seen in the office of the psychiatrist—the neuroses.

Studies of the Process of Change

Clinical trials[12] have left little doubt that desensitization is a very effective method for overcoming specific fears. But because the psychotherapeutic interview situation is highly complex, controlled experiments have been needed to find out whether the desensitization procedure per se is responsible for the effects observed. The first rigorous studies were performed by Lang and Lazovik[13] and Lang et al.[14] They found in snake phobias that subjects treated by desensitization showed significantly greater reduction in snake avoidance and reported less fear than either subjects who were untreated or those subjected to a "pseudotherapy" based upon a plausible, vaguely psychoanalytic theory, and that the results were unrelated to suggestibility. The differences were preserved at follow-up. Paul[15] found that psychoanalytically oriented therapists, treating students with severe fears of public speaking, did significantly better with desensitization than they did with their own customary insight therapy or with an "attention-placebo" method (although both of the latter achieved more change than was found in untreated controls).

Several studies have been addressed to the question whether the state of relaxation and systematized scene presentations must *both* be present for desensitization to be effective. Davison,[16] working with snake phobias, and Rachman,[17] with spider phobias, each found that serial scene presentations alone and relaxation alone reduced fear to some extent, but significantly less than the combination. In a clinical setting Moore[18] treated cases of asthma by three schedules: relaxation only, support and suggestion with relaxation, and systematic desensitization. Both after treatment and at follow-up, the effects of desensitization were the most marked, its superiority measured by maximum peak flow of inspired air being significant at the level of 0.001.

For years we leaned largely on Jacobson's[8] observations of the autonomic effects of muscle relaxation. These have now been supported and extended by several careful investigations. Paul[19] showed that muscle relaxation elicits effects opposite to those characteristic of anxiety on heart rate, respiratory rate, and skin conductance, most markedly if the relaxation follows relaxation training, but also significantly if it is induced by hypnotic suggestion or by simple instructions to relax. Paul[20] furthermore demonstrated that autonomic arousal by a stressful stimulus decreases to the extent that previous relaxation has had contrary-to-anxiety effects. In other words, the greater the basal "calmness," the less anxiety a given stimulus elicits. Van Egeren and Feather,[21] in an elaborate psychophysiological study involving skin conductance, heart rate, digital pulse amplitude, and respiratory rate, found that relaxed subjects showed less decrease in skin resistance to verbal stimuli of phobic content than did those who were not relaxed, and in addition that with repetitions of the stimuli, the magnitude of the change progressively lessened further in the relaxed but remained more or less stationary in the unrelaxed. Similarly, in an experiment comparing the effects of presenting hierarchical stimuli in a standardized way to relaxed and to nonrelaxed subjects,[22] a consistent downward trend of the autonomic arousal (galvanic skin response) due to each stimulus was noted across sessions for relaxed, but not for nonrelaxed subjects.

Technical Variants of Desensitization

As noted in the introduction to this article, conventional systematic desensitization is a particular implementation of an experimentally established principle. There is constant research into other possibilities, partly because desensitization is not always practicable and partly because of the need to find still more effective and economical methods.

Desensitization in Groups. Several patients with the same phobia may all be trained to relax and then subjected to desensitization simultaneously. Paul and Shannon[23] and Donner and Guerney[24] have found that, at least with relatively simple phobic material, there is little difference between the effects of group and individual desensitization.

Automated Procedures. Another innovation economizing on therapists' time is the use of mechanical aids. Lang,[25] and Migler and Wolpe[26] have used tape recorders in place of the living therapist to present hierarchical material to phobic patients. A comparative study by Lang et al.[27] indicates that this does not diminish the effectiveness of the procedure. Denholtz[28] has extended the use of tape recorders to flooding and aversive therapy (see below). Budzinsky et al.[29] have reported the use of auditory feedback from electromyographic activity as an aid to relaxation.

Physical Presentation of Phobic Stimuli. A number of subjects, about 15 percent, have no emotional response when imagining situations that disturb them when encountered in actuality. It is then futile to attempt standard desensitization and necessary to present the stimuli substantively. Sometimes pictorial presentation will do. Goldberg and D'Zurilla[30] have overcome fears of injections by the use of slide projections of the stages of activity involved in giving an injection, and Dengrove[31] has used movie film to overcome phobias for bridges. In other cases, one is reduced to exposing the patient to the real situation—relatively easy to do when the fear is of some portable object or animal (e.g., a spider), but inconvenient when the fear is of heights or of open spaces—for then the patient has to be accompanied to the relevant situations in their hierarchical order. An effective though more complex type of reality exposure called *modeling* has been introduced by Bandura.[32] The patient watches a fearless model whose behavior he is gently guided to imitate.

Anxiety-Inhibiting Responses Other Than Relaxation. A certain number of patients either cannot or will not learn muscle relaxation, sometimes because they have a fear of letting go that is triggered by relaxation. It is then necessary to turn to some other anxiety-inhibiting response, of which, fortunately, a considerable number are available. One of the simplest is obtained by weak electrical stimulation of the forearm. Apparently, the internal responses to the electrical pulses inhibit the small amount of anxiety that is aroused by weak phobic stimuli. When the patient signals that he has clearly formed the requested image, two or three pulses are passed into his forearm.[9] Another method of inhibiting anxiety is by the evocation, through imagery, of other emotions that are antagonistic to it. Suitable contexts may be determined by the use of a questionnaire.[33] Stimuli that are disturbing to the patient are presented to him in hierarchical order in the context previously identified—e.g., sexual activity, lying on the beach, skiing.

Other Behavioral Methods for Overcoming Anxiety Habits

The central feature of desensitization methods is the systematic reduction by reciprocal inhibition of the anxiety-evoking power of various stimuli. Reciprocal inhibition also enters into other modes of anxiety reduction that are less systematic and sometimes include other learning processes. The course of life overcomes many neuroses, seemingly by juxtaposing other emotional responses with anxiety-evoking stimuli that are incidentally present, and much the same thing happens in therapeutic transactions of all kinds when fearful words and images come up while the patient is responding with pleasant excitation to the therapist. In addition, there are behavior therapy techniques that depend on arranging for reciprocal inhibition to occur in the life situation—for example, assertive behavior or programmatically delimited sexual behavior.[9]

Tranquilizing drugs have been used in behavior therapy in several ways. Desensitization is accelerated if relaxation is enhanced by intravenous methohexital (Brevital).[34] Miller et al.[35] demonstrated that rats could be rid of a conditioned emotional response (anxiety) if they were exposed to the conditioned stimuli repeatedly under the "protection" of chlorpramazine, but not if exposed without the drug, or if given the drug without the exposure. This observation encouraged some desultory clinical applications,[9] and recently Hussain[36] has reported strikingly rapid improvement in anxiety neuroses following strong and prolonged exposure to the relevant imaginary stimuli under pentobarbital, but no change if the procedure is administered without the drug.

However, favorable effects have often been obtained by others by long-continued elicitation of anxiety responses[37-39] —a procedure nowadays known as *flooding*. A man with acrophobia may be asked to imagine himself looking out of a tenth-floor window for 30 minutes at a stretch, or, if necessary, may be physically conducted and kept there for that period. At present, flooding should be used with hesitation, since controlled studies[40-42] show it to be less effective than systematic desensitization. Moreover, it is an unpleasant method and occasionally makes patients worse instead of better.

Aversion Therapy

This term applies to procedures aimed at breaking unadaptive habits by the use of a strong stimulus to suppress the behavior one wishes to eliminate. For example, in a 9-month infant with persistent vomiting without organic cause Lang and Melamed[43] applied 1-second electric shocks sufficient to be painful, at the start of the vomiting and at 1-second intervals as long as it went on. The vomiting stopped completely by the sixth session. A 6-month follow-up revealed no recurrence, and a normal, healthy child.

Aversion therapy is, for obvious reasons, used sparingly in behavior therapy but clearly has a role. Much of its recent usage has been in the treatment of homosexuality,[44] by a technique in which shock accompanying the projection of a homosexual figure on a screen is switched off at the appearance of an attractive female. This method frequently leads to a lasting reversal to heterosexuality, but it should not be used before the anxiety conditionings that are the rule in homosexuality have been dealt with. Other common targets are fetishes and compulsive behavior. Aversion therapy has also been used for alcoholism but the technique is cumbersome and requires "boosters." A single case study[45] has suggested the possibility of a treatment for addictions that is at least temporarily effective.

Cautela[46] has described an interesting aversion technique in which the imagining of the unwanted behavior is paired with verbally induced aversive responses, such as nausea.

Operant Conditioning

The procedures under this heading are based on experimental paradigms developed by B. F. Skinner and his associates. In general, a habit is strengthened if reward follows the response that expresses it, and weakened if no reward follows. The operant conditioning element in assertive training was pointed out above, but operant conditioning is the sole technique in many other contexts. For example, thumb sucking in young children has been markedly and lastingly reduced by turning off a movie cartoon whenever the child sucks his thumb.[47] Encopresis[48] has been successfully treated by arranging to give candy following defecation, and Kimmel and Kimmel[49] have described a treatment of enuresis nocturna in which the child is rewarded for increasingly long diurnal retention of urine.

In most of the earlier efforts at operant treatment, primary rewards, such as food, were exclusively employed. Recently, there has been increasing use of tokens[1,50] especially in ward treatment programs known as *token economies*. The patient can later use the tokens his behavior has earned him to buy privileges of his own choice.[1,51] The technique has been applied to a wide range of unadaptive behaviors, including "character disorders," [52] delinquency,[53,54] antisocial behavior,[55] and pill taking.[56]

Token economies to modify undesirable classroom behavior were first introduced by O'Leary and Becker.[57] During a 2-month token period they reduced disruptive behavior (talking, noise, pushing, eating) by about 80 percent. Several similar studies have since been reported.[58-60] In a controlled comparison in which the dependent measures were task attention and achievement in reading and arithmetic, Hewett et al.[61] found significantly more improvement in the token-receiving class. An excellent text for those interested in applying token and other operant programs to children's problems has been provided by Patterson and Guillion.[62]

Tokens may also be used to modify complex individual interractions. Stuart[63] has designed a program that has been very effective in restoring harmony in disordered marriages. Each partner lists the behavior changes desired in the other. The partners are assisted by the therapist in recapturing reciprocity in their interractions. Tokens are handed from one to the other according to the number of times specified behavior has been earned. It is essential, in using this technique, to emphasize to the subjects that "personality" is known and expressed only through behavior and does not subsist in some "deep" and immutable core. In Stuart's original article all of five marriages were reported to have been successfully restored.

Patterson and Gullion also make extensive use of social reinforcers—the habit-strengthening effects upon the subject of someone in his environment attending, nodding, smiling, applauding, and in various verbal ways expressing approval upon the performance of specified behavior. Such reinforcement, which is "naturally" available in the environment, has played an increasing part in the procedures of child behavior therapists.[64-68]

Concluding Remarks

The various applications of learning principles that behavior therapy embodies have been tested by a volume of research that is unique in the psychotherapeutic field.[11] This work has supported the presumption that for those behaviors of psychiatric concern that are learned, the key lies in the utilization of learning principles. Of especial practical significance is the finding of rapid recovery of most cases of neurosis (in about 30 sessions on the average), without subsequent relapse or symptom substitution.[7]

Nevertheless, many criticisms have been leveled at this approach. The most widely quoted critique, by Breger and McGaugh,[69] raises a variety of objections—*inter alia,* that behavior therapy is limited to "symptom removal," that it is too mechanical, and that "modern learning theory," upon which it is supposed to be based, does not exist. Most of these criticisms are based on misconceptions of behavior therapy; for example, it is not based upon "learning theory" but upon experimental paradigms. Breger and McGaugh have been answered in detail by Rachman and Eysenck[70] and by Wiest.[71] More recent critiques by Weitzman[72] and Costello[73] have also been answered by Wolpe.[74] This is not to contend that the theory or the practice of behavior therapy is without blemish. In fact, difficulties abound, but not in the directions suggested by these critics.

The greatest problem at present is the provision of suitable training facilities for psychiatrists and clinical psychologists who would like to become proficient in behavior therapy procedures. In only a handful of university departments is adequate training available,[75] but their number is only slowly increasing. In the meantime, the deficiency is to some extent being compensated for by a number of journals devoted to the topic—*Behavior Research and Therapy*, *The Journal of Behavior Therapy and Experimental Psychiatry*, *Behavior Therapy*, and *The Journal of Applied Behavior Analysis*.

REFERENCES

1. Ayllon, T., and Azrin, N. H.: The Token Economy: A Motivational System for Therapy and Rehabilitation. New York, Appleton-Century-Crofts, 1968.
2. Schaffer, H. H., and Martin, P. L.: Behavioral Therapy. New York, McGraw-Hill Book Co., Inc., 1969.
3. Pavlov, I.: Conditioned Reflexes and Psychiatry. Trans. by W. H. Gantt. New York, International Publications, 1941.
4. Anderson, O. D., and Parmenter, R.: A Long Term Study of the Experimental Neurosis in the Sheep and Dog. Psychosom. Med. Monogr. 2, Nos. 3 and 4, 1941.
5. Masserman, J. H.: Behavior and Neurosis. Chicago, University of Chicago Press, 1943.
6. Wolpe, J.: Experimental Neurosis as Learned Behavior. Brit. J. Psychol. 43:243-268, 1952.
7. Wolpe, J.: Psychotherapy by Reciprocal Inhibition. Stanford, Calif., Stanford University Press, 1958.
8. Jacobson, E.: Progressive Relaxation. Chicago, University of Chicago Press, 1938.
9. Wolpe, J.: The Practice of Behavior Therapy. New York, Pergamon Press, 1969.
10. Wolpe, J.: Behavior Therapy in Complex Neurotic States. Brit. J. Psychiat. 110:28-34, 1964.
11. Krasner, L.: Behavior Therapy. Ann. Rev. Psychol. 22:483-532, 1971.
12. Wolpe, J.: The Systematic Desensitization Treatment of Neuroses. J. Nerv. Ment. Dis. 132:189-203, 1961.
13. Lang, P. J., and Lazovik, A. D.: The Experimental Desensitization of a Phobia. J. Abnorm. Soc. Psychol. 66:519-525, 1963.
14. Lang, P. J., Lazovik, A. D., and Reynolds, D. J.: Desensitization, Suggestibility, and Pseudotherapy. J. Abnorm. Psychol. 70:395-402, 1965.
15. Paul, G. L.: Insight Versus Desensitization in Psychotherapy: An Experiment in Anxiety Reduction. Stanford, Calif., Stanford University Press, 1966.
16. Davison, G. C.: The Influence of Systematic Desensitization, Relaxation and Graded Exposure to Imaginal Aversive Stimuli on the Modification of Phobic Behavior. Stanford, Calif., Unpublished Doctoral Dissertation, 1965.
17. Rachman, S.: Studies in Desensitization: I. The Separate Effects of Relaxation and Desensitization. Behav. Res. Ther. 3:245-251, 1965.
18. Moore, N.: Behavior Therapy in Bronchial Asthma: A Controlled Study. J. Psychosom. Res. 9:257-276, 1965.
19. Paul, G. L.: Physiological Effects of Relaxation Training and Hypnotic Suggestion. J. Abnorm. Psychol. 74:425-437, 1969.
20. Paul, G. L.: Inhibition of Physiological Response to Stressful Imagery by Relaxation Training and Hypnotically Suggested Relaxation. Behav. Res. Ther. 7:249-256, 1969.

21. Van Egeren, L. F., and Feather, S. W.: Psychophysiology of Systematic Desensitization: I. Imagery, Relaxation, Counterconditioning and Extinction. Psychophysiol. (in press).
22. Wolpe, J., and Flood, J.: The Effect of Relaxation on the Galvanic Skin Response to Repeated Phobic Stimuli in Ascending Order. J. Behav. Ther. Exp. Psychiat. 1:195-200, 1970.
23. Paul, G. L., and Shannon, D. T.: Treatment of Anxiety Through Systematic Desensitization in Therapy Groups. J. Abnorm. Psychol. 71:124-135, 1966.
24. Donner, L., and Guerney, B. G., Jr.: Automated Group Desensitization for Test Anxiety. Behav. Res. Ther. 7:1-13, 1969.
25. Lang, P. J.: Personal Communication, 1966.
26. Migler, B., and Wolpe, J.: Automated Desensitization: A Case Report. Behav. Res. Ther. 5:133-135, 1967.
27. Lang, P. J., Melamed, B. G., and Hart, J.: A Psychophysiological Analysis of Fear Modification Using an Automated Desensitization Procedure. J. Abnorm. Psychol. 76:221-234, 1970.
28. Denholtz, M.: The Use of Tape Recordings Between Therapy Sessions. J. Behav. Ther. Exp. Psychiat. 1:139-143, 1970.
29. Budzinsky, T., Stoyva, J., and Adler, C.: Feedback-Induced Muscle Relaxation: Application to Tension Headache. J. Behav. Ther. Exp. Psychiat. 1:205-211, 1970.
30. Goldberg, J., and D'Zurilla, T. G.: Demonstration of Slide Projection as an Alternative to Imaginal Stimulus Presentation in Systematic Desensitization Therapy. Psychol. Rep. 23:527-533, 1968.
31. Dengrove, E.: Personal Communication, 1968.
32. Bandura, A.: Principles of Behavior Modification. New York, Holt, Rinehart, and Winston, 1969.
33. Cautela, J., and Kastenbaum, R.: A Reinforcement Survey Schedule for Use in Therapy, Training and Research. Psychol. Rep. 20:1115-1130, 1967.
34. Brady, J. P.: Brevital-Relaxation Treatment of Frigidity. Behav. Res. Ther. 4:71-77, 1966.
35. Miller, N. E., Murphy, J. V., and Mirsky, I. A.: Persistent Effects of Chlorpromazine on Extinction of an Avoidance Response. Arch. Neurol. Psychiat. 78:526, 1957.
36. Hussain, M. Z.: Desensitization and Flooding (Implosion) in Treatment of Phobias. Amer. J. Psychiat. 127:1509-1514, 1971.
37. Malleson, N.: Panic and Phobia. Lancet. 1:225-227, 1959.
38. Stampfl, T. G., and Levis, D. J.: Essentials of Implosive Therapy: A Learning-Theory-Based Psychodynamic Behavioral Therapy. J. Abnorm. Psychol. 72:496-503, 1967.
39. Watson, J. P., and Marks, I. M.: Relevant and Irrelevant Fear in Flooding—A Crossover Study of Phobic Patients. Behav. Ther. 2:275-293, 1971.
40. Willis, R. W., and Edwards, J. A.: A Study of the Comparative Effectiveness of the Systematic Desensitization and Implosive Therapy. Behav. Res. Ther. 7:387-395, 1969.
41. DeMoor, W.: Systematic Desensitization Versus Prolonged High Intensity Stimulation (Flooding). J. Behav. Ther. Exp. Psychiat. 1:45-52, 1970.
42. Mealia, W. L., and Nawas, M. M.: The Comparative Effectiveness of Systematic Desensitization and Implosive Therapy in the Treatment of Snake Phobia. J. Behav. Ther. Exp. Psychiat. 2:85-94, 1971.
43. Lang, P. J., and Melamed, B. G.: Avoidance Conditioning Therapy of an Infant with Chronic Ruminative Vomiting. J. Abnorm. Psychol. 74:1-8, 1969.

44. Feldman, M. P., and MacCullogh, M. J.: Aversion Therapy in the Management of Homosexuals. Brit. Med. J. 1:594-598, 1967.
45. Wolpe, J.: Conditioned Inhibition of Craving in Drug Addiction: A Pilot Experiment. Behav. Res. Ther. 2:285-289, 1965.
46. Cautela, J. R.: Covert Sensitization. Psychol. Rec. 20:459-468, 1967.
47. Baer, D. M.: Laboratory Control of Thumbsucking by Withdrawal and Re-presentation of Reinforcement. J. Exp. Anal. Behav. 5:525-528, 1962.
48. Neale, D. H.: Behavior Therapy and Encopresis in Children. Behav. Res. Ther. 1:139-149, 1963.
49. Kimmel, H. D., and Kimmel, E.: An Instrumental Conditioning Method for the Treatment of Enuresis. J. Behav. Ther. Exp. Psychiat. 1:121-123, 1970.
50. Staats, A. W., Staats, C. K., Schutz, R. E., and Wolf, M. M.: The Conditioning of Textual Responses Using "Extrinsic" Reinforcers. J. Exp. Anal. Behav. 5:33-40, 1962.
51. Lloyd, K. E., and Garlington, W. K.: Weekly Variations in Performance on a Token Economy Psychiatric Ward. Behav. Res. Ther. 6:407-410, 1968.
52. Colman, A. D., and Baker, S. L.: Utilization of an Operant Conditioning Model for the Treatment of Character and Behavior Disorders in a Military Setting. Amer. J. Psychiat. 125:1395-1403, 1969.
53. Cohen, H. L.: Educational Therapy: The Design of Learning Environments. In: Schlein, J. M. (Ed.), Research in Psychotherapy. Washington, D.C., American Psychological Association, 1968.
54. Fineman, K. R.: An Operant Conditioning Program in a Juvenile Detention Facility. Psychol. Rep. 22:1119-1120, 1968.
55. Burchard, J. D.: Systematic Socialization: A Programmed Environment for the Habilitation of Anti-social Retardates. Psychol. Rec. 17:461-476, 1967.
56. Parrino, J. J., George, L., and Daniels, A. C.: Token Control of Pill-Taking Behavior in a Psychiatric Ward. J. Behav. Ther. Exp. Psychiat., 1971. (in press).
57. O'Leary, K. D., and Becker, W. C.: Behavior Modification of an Adjustment Class: A Token Reinforcement Program. Exceptional Child. 33:637-642, 1967.
58. Patterson, G. R.: Behavioral Intervention Procedures in the Classroom and the Home. In: Bergin, A. E., and Garfield, S. L. (Eds.), Handbook of Psychotherapy and Behavior Change. New York, Wiley, 1970.
59. Walker, H. M., Mattson, R. H., and Buckley, N. K.: Special Class Placement as a Treatment Alternative for Deviant Behavior in Children. In: Benson, F. A. M. (Ed.), Modifying Deviant Social Behaviors in Various Classroom Settings. Monogr. No. 1. Oregon, Dept. of Special Education, University of Oregon, 1969.
60. Meichenbaum, D. H., Bowers, K. S., and Ross, R. R.: Modification of Classroom Behavior of Institutionalized Female Adolescent Offenders. Behav. Res. Ther. 6:343-353, 1968.
61. Hewett, F. M., Taylor, F. D., and Artuso, A. A.: The Santa Monica Project: Evaluation of an Engineered Classroom Design with Emotionally Disturbed Children. J. Coun. Except. Child. 35:523-529, 1969.
62.. Patterson, G. R., and Gullion, M. E.: Living with Children: New Methods for Parents and Teachers. Champaign, Ill., Research Press, 1968.
63. Stuart, R. B.: Operant-Interpersonal Treatment for Marital Discord. J. Consult. Clin. Psychol. 33:675-682, 1969.
64. Ferster, C. B., and Simons, J.: Behavior Therapy with Children. Psychol. Rec. 16:65-71, 1966.

65. Guerney, B. G. (Ed.): Psychotherapeutic Agents: New Roles for Nonprofessionals, Parents and Teachers. New York, Holt, Rinehart and Winston, 1969.

66. Patterson, G. R., McNeal, S., Hawkins, N., and Phelps, R.: Reprogramming the Social Environment. J. Child. Psychol. Psychiat. 8:181-195, 1967.

67. Wahler, R. G.: Oppositional Children: A Quest for Parental Reinforcement Control. J. Appl. Behav. Anal. 2:159-170, 1969.

68. Wahler, R. G., and Cormier, Wm. H.: The Ecological Interview: A First Step in Out-Patient Child Behavior Therapy. J. Behav. Ther. Exp. Psychiat. 1:279-289, 1970.

69. Breger, L., and McGaugh, J. L.: A Critique and Reformulation of "Learning Theory" Approaches to Psychotherapy and Neurosis. Psychol Bull. 63:335-358, 1965.

70. Rachman, S., and Eysenck, H. J.: Reply to a "Critique and Reformulation" of Behavior Therapy. Psychol. Bull. 65:165-169, 1966.

71. Wiest, W. M.: Some Recent Criticisms of Behaviorism and Learning Theory. Psychol. Bull. 67:214-225, 1967.

72. Weitzman, B.: Behavior Therapy and Psychotherapy. Psychol. Rev. 74: 300-317, 1967.

73. Costello, C. G.: Dissimilarities Between Conditioned Avoidance Responses and Phobias. Psychol. Rev. 77:250-254, 1970.

74. Wolpe, J.: The Behavioristic Conception of Neurosis: A Reply to Two Critics. Psychol. Rev. 78:341-343, 1971.

75. Edwards, N. B.: Behavior Therapy Training in the United States. J. Behav. Ther. Exp. Psychiat. 1:179-181, 1970.

Aversion Therapy of Homosexuality

by Neil McConaghy, M.D., D.P.M.

In evaluating the efficacy of the various treatments of homosexuality the same questions require answering as with the investigation of any psychiatric therapy. These are: What are the aims of treatment? Can the achievement of these aims be attributed to the specific effects of the treatment? How can the achievement of different aims by various treatments be compared?

In studies utilizing either relationship psychotherapy or aversion therapy for homosexual patients, a common aim has been that the subjects adopt heterosexual patterns of behavior. Other aims have varied, e.g., to what extent should the patients cease homosexual behaviour, and should they obtain "insight" into the postulated origins of their homosexuality? As regards the achievement of the common aim, psychotherapy and aversion therapy have not been shown to differ significantly. Woodward[16] reported that 36 percent and Bieber[2] that 27 percent of their homosexual patients became exclusively heterosexual following psychotherapy; MacCulloch and Feldman[8] reported a similar response in 33 percent of their subjects following aversion therapy. The last authors also stated that 58 percent became heterosexual as judged by the Kinsey scale.[7] Mayerson and Lief,[9] using a similarly less rigorous definition of heterosexuality, concluded that 50 percent of their group achieved this state following psychotherapy. Freund[6] considered that 18 percent of the patients he treated showed a satisfactory response in that they had heterosexual intercourse regularly for several years following aversion therapy. He was the only one of these workers to follow up his subjects for such a long period of time, and the only one to report that some of his patients at later interviews admitted they had lied about their degree of response earlier.

Conclusions concerning the efficacy of the two forms of therapy have varied considerably. Coates[4] considered that psychotherapy was superior, whereas MacCulloch and Feldman[8] claimed the advantage for their form of behavior therapy. Freund[6] and Bieber[3] decided the results of both were similar, in respect to changing sexual behavior. As none of the groups treated can be accepted as comparable, in the absence of data from controlled trials evaluating the two forms of therapy, such conclusions are likely to continue to vary.

Regarding the degree to which the results reported above can be attributed to the specific effects of the treatment, uncertainty must again prevail. Most psychiatrists have had the experience of seeing patients or other acquaintances cease homosexual or other deviant forms of behavior under the influence of religious beliefs or guilt-provoking pressures and at times become unaware of the existence of the feelings that led to the deviant behavior. To the extent the above therapies produce changes in patients' conscious feelings and sexual activity, these therapies could be operating in similar ways, without producing any actual change in the strength of the patients' homosexual or heterosexual drives.

In an attempt to overcome this problem a series of studies were carried out to determine whether an objective technique could be developed which measured the strength of such sexual drives, and if so, whether such a technique could be used to demonstrate changes due to treatment. Facilities were not available for the psychotherapeutic treatment of a large series of homosexual patients, and aversion therapy alone was studied. It was additionally decided to investigate the mode of action of this therapy—in particular to determine if it acted by setting up conditioned reflexes, as has been generally accepted.[5]

Measuring Sexual Orientation

The objective measure investigated was the recording of changes in the subject's penile volume while he watched a travelogue-type moving film. At approximately 1-minute intervals there were inserted into the film 10 segments of 10-second shots of an orange circle followed by 10-second shots of nude young women, alternating with 10 10-second shots of a blue triangle followed by 10-second shots of nude young men. The sexual orientation of the subject was determined by measuring the 10 penile volume changes to the shots of women and the 10 to shots of men and testing the significance of the difference between the two groups of 10 scores using the Mann-Whitney U test.[10]

As a control group 11 medical students who were confident of their heterosexual orientation volunteered to undergo this film assessment. All showed greater penile volume increase to the pictures of women, 10 to a statistically significant extent. An unexpected finding was that these subjects commonly showed a penile volume decrease to pictures of the males. Penile volume increases to the orange circles preceding the female nudes and decreases to the blue triangles preceding the male nudes occurred as conditioned responses.[13] Similar results were obtained in a larger study investigating 60 psychology student volunteers.[1]

Comparison of Apomorphine Aversion and Aversion-Relief Therapy

The initial aversion treatment study investigated the response of 40 homosexual patients. As expected, in the film assessment they tended to show penile volume increases to the pictures of the males, decreases to those of the females, and appropriate conditioned responses to the preceding circles and triangles. The conditioned responses were used to provide a measure of each of the homosexual subjects' ability to set up conditioned responses—his so-called conditionability.

The primary aim of the first treatment study was to compare the efficacy of two forms of aversion treatment, using as measures of response both the patients' subjective reports of change in sexual feelings and behavior and the changes in penile volume reactions to the shots of male and female nudes. As stated earlier, the aversion therapies are widely considered to act by setting up conditioned responses. A secondary aim was to obtain evidence for or against this theory by examining the relationship between each subject's ability to respond to aversion therapy and his ability to set up conditioned responses in the sexual orientation film assessment. In the first study the two treatments compared were apomorphine aversion and aversion relief. Both methods have been claimed to be effective in treating homosexuality.[6,15]

With apomorphine aversion, the subject was initially given a subcutaneous injection of 1.5 mg. of apomorphine. After a variable interval, usually about 8 minutes, he commenced to feel nauseated. Severe nausea lasting 10 minutes without vomiting was aimed for and the dose constantly adjusted throughout treatment to maintain this response. The patient timed the onset of the nausea and one minute prior to its expected onset switched on a slide projector and viewed a slide of a nude or seminude male which he found sexually exciting. Prior to the nausea reaching its maximum he turned off the projector. Twenty-eight such treatment sessions were administered at two-hourly periods over five days, each patient being admitted to the hospital for the five days.

With aversion-relief therapy, for each patient 14 slides were made of words and phrases considered by the patient to be evocative of aspects of homosexuality which he found exciting. These slides were projected at 10-second intervals. The patient read each one aloud. Immediately after he finished reading he received a painful electric shock through electrodes attached to the fingertips. Following the 14 slides, one was projected which related to aspects of normal sexuality. This was left on for 40 seconds and not accompanied by a shock. The appearance of this slide produced a sense of relief as the patient learned it would not be accompanied by a shock. In one treatment session this procedure was carried out five times, with intervals of 2½ minutes intervening. Three treatment sessions were given daily for 5 consecutive days during which the patients were hospitalized. Hence each patient received a total of 1050 shocks during treatment.

Subjects. Forty persons conscious of homosexual feeling who wished to have this reduced and who were not overtly psychotic were accepted for treatment. Eighteen had been arrested for homosexual behavior, eight on more than one occasion. Legal action had led to 6 of the 18 coming for treatment, the other 12 no longer being under any form of constraint. Ten patients were married and 20 considered they were sexually aroused by women or had been in the past, four stating that their heterosexual interest was greater than their homosexual interest. These four had all been arrested for homosexual behavior—one on three occasions. Thirty-eight had had homosexual relations with a number of partners. Two had had no overt homosexual experience since adolescence; one of these was distressed by his strong feelings of attraction to other men, the other by homosexual sadistic fantasies.

Method. The 40 patients were randomly allocated to two groups of 20, one group to receive immediate treatment, one delayed treatment. Each group of 20 was further randomly allocated to two groups of 10, one group to receive apomorphine, the other aversion-relief therapy. The immediate treatment group viewed the sexual orientation assessment film immediately prior to treatment and again 3 weeks later. The delayed-treatment group viewed the film 3 weeks prior to treatment as well as on these two occasions. This enabled any changes occurring in the immediately treated group after treatment to be compared with changes occurring over the same period of time, without treatment, in the delayed-treatment group. At three weeks following treatment the patients were also interviewed about change in sexual feelings and behavior.

Results. In the delayed-treatment group there was no significant change in penile volume responses in the film assessment without treatment intervening. Following treatment, the immediate treatment group showed significantly less penile volume increase to the pictures of nude men, compared to their response prior to treatment. As regards the penile volume response to the pictures of women, those patients who showed penile volume decrease to these pictures before treatment showed significantly less decrease following treatment. There was no change in the responses of those patients who before treatment showed no change or penile volume increase to these pictures. The changes in penile volume to pictures of men and women were still present without any weakening at follow-up a year later.

The patients also reported reduction in their homosexual and increase in their heterosexual feelings and behavior. The reported reduction in homosexuality was greater at 2 weeks than at 1 year following treatment; the reverse was true in respect to heterosexuality. These reported changes in sexual feelings correlated significantly with the changes to the sexual orientation film at 1-year follow-up, but not at 2 weeks following treatment. It was concluded that the reported changes at 1 year were more reliable than those at 2 weeks, the longer time allowing the patients to assess their feelings more accurately.

At 1 year following treatment, approximately half the patients reported reduction in homosexual feelings and a half—not necessarily the same patients—an increase in heterosexual feelings. A quarter reported they had ceased homosexual behaviour and a quarter—not necessarily the same—that they had commenced or increased the frequency of heterosexual intercourse. However, all patients were still aware of some degree of homosexual feelings. There were no significant differences in the results of the two treatments, either in changes to the film assessment or in reported sexual feelings and behavior. There was no consistent relationship between each subject's outcome with treatment and his conditionability as measured by the amplitude of his conditioned responses in the film assessment. This study has been reported in greater detail elsewhere.[11,12]

Comparison of Apomorphine Aversion and Avoidance Conditioning

MacCulloch and Feldman[8] reported a much better outcome, at least in terms of complete loss of homosexual feeling, in patients treated with an aversive technique using avoidance learning. With this technique, the patient viewed the slide of a male and was instructed to leave it on as long as he found it attractive. After 8 seconds he commenced to receive an electric shock if he had not removed the slide by means of a hand switch with which he was provided. The shock continued until he removed the slide. Once he avoided the shock three times in succession, by switching the male slide off before 8 seconds had elapsed, he was placed on a schedule of reinforcement. On one-third of the trials he could still switch the slide off whenever he wished; on another third he could switch off the slide after a variable delay; and on the final third he could not switch the slide off until after he received a shock. On some occasions following the removal of the male slide and cessation of the shock, the slide of a woman was shown—with the expectation that this might increase heterosexual feeling.

This aversive technique was compared with apomorphine aversion in a further study, similar in design to the initial one, comparing apomorphine aversion with aversion-relief. The subjects were approximately comparable to those of the first study. Avoidance conditioning was given in 14 sessions of treatment over 5 days. During each session the male slide was shown 30 times. The apomorphine treatment procedure was basically unchanged.[14] The aims were to attempt to replicate the findings of MacCulloch and Feldman as to the greater efficacy of avoidance learning and to replicate the findings of the first study as to the changes following apomorphine aversion.

Only the second aim was realized. There was no significant difference in outcome with the two treatments. Both treatments produced a similar degree of reduction in homosexuality as indicated by the patients' subjective reports and by the changes in their response to the sexual assessment film. There was again a significant correlation between these two measures of outcome. No weakening in the change in response to the sexual assessment film occurred at follow-up 6 months later. There was no consistent relationship between response to treatment and the subjects as measured in the film assessment.

Most subjects are unaware of the changes in penile volume measured in the sexual assessment. It would seem unlikely that these changes could be under conscious control. Hence their modification with treatment and the correlated reduction in reported homosexual feeling would appear to be valid indicators that the treatment is at least to some extent effective. The disconcerting finding of the two studies is that three widely different aversive techniques have produced essentially the same results. Feldman and MacCulloch stated they designed the elaborate technique of avoidance learning to fully exploit the many thousands of experiments on animal and human learning with the expectation that it would prove a much more effective therapy. If the aversion therapies act by setting up conditioned responses, this application of learning principles to obtain better conditioning must result in a more effective therapy. That it did not suggests strongly that these therapies do not act in this way. This is further suggested by the fact that there was no consistent relationship between a patient's ability to set up conditioned responses in the assessment film and his degree of response to aversion therapy.

Comparison of Classical, Avoidance, and Backward Conditioning

To investigate this further, a third study was carried out. A similar design was followed to the previous ones, except that three aversive techniques were compared—avoidance learning, classical conditioning, and backward conditioning. With classical conditioning, 10 to 15 slides of nude or seminude males to which the patient showed and felt a significant sexual response were selected. Three of these slides were shown to the patient for 10 seconds in each treatment session. Overlapping and continuing beyond the last second of exposure of each slide, a shock of 2 seconds' duration was administered, of an intensity as high as the patient could tolerate. The three slides were shown at intervals of approximately 4 minutes. The patient received 14 such sessions of treatment over 5 days.

With the backward conditioning procedure the patient received a 1-second shock of the same order of unpleasantness as that used in the avoidance learning procedure. A half second after the shock terminated he was shown for 4 seconds the slide of a male to which he was sexually responsive. Two seconds later either he was shown a slide of a nude or seminude girl or the screen was left blank for 16 seconds. After a further half second he again received the shock which preceded the male slide. This sequence was followed 30 times in each treatment session. The patient received 14 such sessions of treatment over 5 days. The procedure was designed to expose the patient to slides of men and women and to a series of shocks for approximately the same duration as with the avoidance procedure. The major variable altered was the relationship of the stimuli. With the backward procedure the unconditioned stimulus—the shock—preceded rather than followed the conditioned stimulus—the slide of the male. Backward conditioning has been widely found to produce minimal if any stable conditioned responses. Hence, if aversion therapy acts by setting up such responses, it would be expected that this form of treatment would be significantly less effective than avoidance or classical conditioning.

Another variable investigated was the effect of booster treatment. Each patient returned for follow-up film and clinical assessment 3 weeks after termination of treatment. Following these, he was given a session of treatment similar to that he had received previously. He continued to return monthly for such booster treatments for 6 months. He then had a film assessment and received the final booster. After a further 6 months he was interviewed to obtain his reported response at that time. In the first two studies no evidence of weakening in response to aversion treatment occurred over the follow-up period, as measured by the changes in penile volume to pictures of men and women. If aversion therapy acts by setting up conditioned responses, such weakening should occur by the process of extinction, and booster treatment should prevent this weakening, at least in part.

Again all three treatment procedures produced changes in the patients' reported feelings and behavior and in their penile volume responses to the movie shots of men and women comparable to the changes in the first two studies. There were no significant differences in the efficacy of the three treatments, nor did this efficacy appear to be increased by the monthly booster treatments.

Clinical Relevance

The studies carried out indicate that 6 to 12 months following aversion treatment about half the patients report an increase in heterosexual feeling and a decrease in homosexual feeling. A quarter have ceased homosexual activity and a quarter have commenced or increased the frequency of heterosexual intercourse. These changes are paralleled by a decrease in the patients' penile volume response to movie films of nude males, a change which does not appear to be under conscious control. Furthermore, those patients who show penile volume decreases to pictures of women have these significantly reduced following treatment. As all patients were unaware that they showed these penile volume decreases, it seems unlikely that their reduction can be due to the suggestion effects of aversion therapy and argues that a change in the strength of sexual feelings is produced by this treatment. However, techniques of aversion therapy which should maximize conditioning are no more effective than those which should minimize it. It would seem that aversion therapy does not act by producing conditioned responses.

The immediate relevance of these studies to the clinician who wishes to use aversion therapy in the treatment of homosexuality is that it appears unnecessary to use elaborate equipment or treatment procedures. A form of classical conditioning similar to that used in the third study would seem easiest to use. Though, in the studies reported, treatments involving showing pictures of girls did not result in more heterosexual behavior by the patients, there was a trend for more heterosexual feelings to be reported, at least in the first weeks following treatment. It would seem worthwhile to incorporate pictures of girls also.

These studies provide no data on the ideal frequency of treatment, though they indicate that booster treatments are unnecessary if a series of treatments are given intensively over 5 days. However other clinicians using aversion therapy with homosexual patients in office practice have informed the author that they have obtained results which appeared comparable to those obtained in these studies, with treatments given in weekly sessions over a few months. This would not seem surprising in view of the present finding that the efficacy of treatment remained unaffected by grossly manipulating variables which theoretically should be much more important. Until further data become available the clinician can plan the course of aversion treatment with the primary determinants being his and his patient's convenience.

A reasonable procedure would be for the patient to select about 10 slides each of nude adolescent and young men and women to which he felt a sexual response. In each session of treatment three male slides would be shown for 10 seconds, the patient receiving a 2-second shock commencing during the last second of exposure of the male slide. The level of shock should be as unpleasant as the patient will tolerate. Following the shock a slide of a woman would be shown for 20 seconds. Variable intervals of 3 to 5 minutes would be left between showing the three sets of male and female slides. Such sessions of treatment would be given three or more times in the first week and gradually reduced in frequency over the following few months.

Treatment additional to aversion therapy was avoided in the above studies. Of course, a supportive psychotherapeutic attitude is necessary, if not purely on humanitarian grounds, then at least so that the relationship with the therapist is such that it will encourage the patient to continue treatment. Patients who are anxious about sexual involvements with women could be expected to benefit from desensitization therapy in addition. However, the author has not had significant success when he has used this in patients who wished to continue treatment after final follow-up. Systematic study of this treatment both in comparison with and in addition to aversion therapy is indicated.

Adverse psychiatric reactions occurred in less than 10 percent of patients following aversion therapy, when they took the form of depressive or, more rarely, anxiety symptoms. Similar symptoms had occurred in the patients prior to treatment and the author did not consider they were "symptom substitutions." In fact, they were more likely to occur in patients who had failed to respond to treatment.

As to the selection of patients, obviously psychopathic patients do not persist with treatment, nor do many patients who come in a crisis situation. It is best to delay treatment in the latter group until they have a better understanding of their feelings. This of course also applies to patients who are depressed, when their wish for treatment may be motivated by the associated guilt. The author did not treat patients who were overtly psychotic. It has been reported[8] that patients over 30 years old do not respond as well to aversion therapy. In the author's experience they are less likely to completely cease homosexual activity and to initiate heterosexual intercourse. However, they report reduction in their homosexual feelings and behavior as commonly as do younger subjects. This older group of patients are more likely to indulge in illegal activities, such as making sexual contacts in public lavatories, often in an apparently compulsive manner. Reduction in homosexual drive appears to give them more control so they are able to continue their homosexual behavior without being subject to arrest. Many of these older and some of the younger patients state they appreciate the freedom from the continual preoccupation with homosexual thoughts which was present prior to aversion therapy. It would seem to the author that reduction of homosexual feelings without increased heterosexual feelings and behavior, though not an ideal treatment response, may still be a worthwhile one. In *The Republic* Plato said: "Old age has a great sense of calm and relaxation. When the passions have relaxed their hold you have escaped, not from one master, but from many."

Probably few heterosexuals would welcome the sense of calm and relaxation which was won by a loss of sexual passion, but this may not be so for many people whose deviant drives force them to behave in ways which are likely to result in severe social and legal sanctions.

Acknowledgments

The National Health and Medical Research Council of Australia is thanked for providing a grant enabling these studies to be carried out.

REFERENCES

1. Barr, R. F., and McConaghy, N.: Penile Volume Responses to Appetitive and Aversive Stimuli in Relation to Sexual Orientation and Conditioning Performance. Brit. J. Psychiat. 119:377-383, 1971.
2. Bieber, I.: Homosexuality. New York, Basic Books, Inc., 1962.
3. Bieber, I.: Aversion Therapy of Homosexuals. Brit. Med. J. 2:372, 1967.
4. Coates, S.: Clinical Psychology in Sexual Deviation. In: Rosen, I. (Ed.), The Pathology and Treatment of Sexual Deviation. New York, Oxford University Press, 1964.
5. Feldman, M. P., and MacCulloch, M. J.: The Application of Anticipatory Avoidance Learning to the Treatment of Homosexuality. I. Theory, Technique and Preliminary Results. Behav. Res. Ther. 2:165-183, 1965.

6. Freund, K.: Some Problems in the Treatment of Homosexuality. In: Eysenck, H. J. (Ed.), Behaviour Therapy and the Neuroses. London, Pergamon Press, 1960.

7. Kinsey, A. C., Pomeroy, W. B., and Martin, C. E.: Sexual Behavior in the Human Male. Philadelphia, W. B. Saunders Company, 1948.

8. MacCulloch, H. J., and Feldman, M. P.: Aversion Therapy in Management of 43 Homosexuals. Brit. Med. J. 1:594-597, 1967.

9. Mayerson, P., and Lief, H. I.: Psychotherapy of Homoxexuals: A Follow-up Study of Nineteen Cases. In: Marmor, J. (Ed.), Sexual Inversion. New York, Basic Books, Inc., 1965.

10. McConaghy, N.: Penile Volume Change to Moving Pictures of Male and Female Nudes in Heterosexual and Homosexual Males. Behav. Res. Ther. 5:43-48, 1967.

11. McConaghy, N.: Subjective and Penile Plethysmograph Responses Following Aversion-Relief and Apomorphine Aversion Therapy for Homosexual Impulses. Brit. J. Psychiat. 115:723-730, 1969.

12. McConaghy, N.: Subjective and Penile Plethysmograph Responses at Two Weeks and One Year Following Aversion-Relief and Apomorphine Aversion Therapy for Homosexual Impulses. Brit. J. Psychiat. 117:555-561, 1970.

13. McConaghy, N.: Penile Response Conditioning and Its Relationship to Aversion Therapy in Homosexuals. Behav. Ther. 1:213-221, 1970.

14. McConaghy, N., Proctor, D., and Barr, R.: Subjective and Penile Plethysmography Responses to Aversion Therapy for Homosexuality: A Partial Replication (to be published), Arch. Sex. Behav.

15. Thorpe, J. G., Schmidt, E., Brown, P. T., and Castell, D.: Aversion-Relief Therapy: A New Method for General Application. Behav. Res. Ther. 2:71-82, 1964.

16. Woodward, M.: The Diagnosis and Treatment of Homosexual Offenders. Brit. J. Delinq. 9:44-59, 1956.

Contributions of Hypnosis to Psychotherapy

by Lewis R. Wolberg, M.D.

Most practitioners who experiment with hypnosis, and seriously attempt to blend it with their habitual techniques, find that it can be productive under certain conditions, even turning the tide from a threatened failure to a therapeutic success.

I wish I could say that hypnosis has been triumphant in all my cases. It has not. I have had my share of disappointments. But the more I have utilized hypnosis over the years, the more respect I have gained for its potentialities. Indeed for me it has continued to be the most important of all the instrumentalities that I have employed in concert with my general therapeutic techniques. Obviously hypnosis must be blended with basic psychotherapeutic procedures because employed in isolation it has limited value (Conn[1]).

How hypnosis works is still a matter of conjecture. In assaying its impact we are confronted with the same confounding variables that envelop all of the psychotherapy. We are slowly beginning to understand some of these variables, but we have not yet been able to expose them completely to the searchlight of scientific exploration (Frank[4]). In psychotherapy we are still balanced precariously on the peak of mounting ambiguities. We do not even yet possess a conceptually valid paradigm around which we can organize our ideas of interpersonal processes. The complexities of chemical, neurophysiological, intrapsychic, spiritual, and social interactions defy description, let alone analysis. We are reduced to accepting the pragmatic proposition that if a method works we should utilize it (Orne[8]). After all we still do not know how electricity operates, but we are constantly employing and enjoying its miracles.

A convenient way of looking at hypnosis is to regard it as a form of communication which expedites a number of healing processes common to all forms of psychotherapy. One of the most important is that hypnosis enhances the multiple roles the therapist must willy-nilly play with his patients as he leads them through the emotional labyrinths of their illness.

Let us outline a few of these roles. A good deal of relief from tension and restoration of homeostasis is generally scored in psychotherapy as a consequence of the placebo influence. Here the therapist, without design or intent, is regarded as the miraculous healer, a *magician*. In the mind of the patient he possesses the means and the wizardry to bring a halt to his suffering and illness. Faith in the therapist's tactics is an important element in all healing processes. It is especially enhanced by the maneuvers of trance induction and utilization (Shapiro[11]).

A second role the psychotherapist assumes is that of *confessor*. Unlocking the door to one's inner burdens unleashes feelings and fears habitually guarded as too reprehensible to reveal. In addition to the immediate and temporary release from tension, there is in such emotional catharsis the added dividend of exposing onself without disguise to an empathic authority. When the expected conventional shock reactions are not forthcoming, the patient usually responds with greater self-tolerance and self-acceptance, and this may register a permanent imprint on his superego. Hypnosis quickly opens up founts of bottled-up emotion owing to its effect on repression. It thus enhances the confessor roles of the therapist.

Suggestion enters into every authority-subject, professional-client relationship (Weitzenhoffer and Sjoberg[13]). As an expert the professional functions wittingly or unwittingly in the role of *demigod* whose pronouncements are subtly absorbed, often without challenge. In hypnosis, suggestibility, as is well known, is greatly enhanced and hence this therapeutic dimension is accordingly magnified.

Perhaps the word *philanthropist* denegrates the fourth role the therapist plays with his patients by virtue of their relationship. The patient projects his hopes for an encounter with an idealized parental figure who will supply him with the understanding and bounties he feels he failed to receive from his own parents. Obviously this unrealistic camouflage is sooner or later swept away when the therapist fails to come up to expectations, but while it lasts the idealization promotes the acceptance of the therapist's theories and practices which will hopefully continue to exert a therapeutic impact when the therapist eventually becomes a mere flesh-and-blood figure. Hypnosis has a remarkable effect on the relationship and even during the first trance session may cut through resistances that would ordinarily delay the essential establishing of rapport. This is especially important in detached and fearful individuals who put up barriers to any kind of closeness and hence obstruct the evolvement of a working alliance.

The fifth role assumed by a productive therapist is that of an *identification model*. Often without awareness the patient's values are recast in the mold of the therapeutic relationship. The patient quickly senses the kind of human being with whom he is dealing from a variety of verbal and nonverbal cues. An amalgamation of the therapist's with his own values occurs gradually, sometimes stirring up conflict. Signs of conflict may not appear in direct form. Value change occurs when the patient works through his need for spurious gratifications inherent in the retention of his neurotic way of life. We assume, of course, that the therapist's values are more realistic and constructive than those of the patient. Hypnosis often elevates the image of the therapist as an idealized authority and expedites his role as an identification model (Dreikurs[3]).

The sixth role of *benefactor* is one that the therapist usually does not deliberately assume, but which may be bestowed on him by a hopeful recipient eager to incorporate palliative subsidies. Even though the patient's incentives may be spurious, the end result can be an incorporation of reinforcements that can shape behavior toward a more healthful adaptation (Dorcus[2]). Once a new behavioral response has been established, or neurotic sequences controlled, certain favorable consequences may occrue to the benefit of the individual, and these positive reinforcers help to maintain accelerated change. There is little question in studying the dreams and associations of subjects in and following a trance that they are inclined to augment the powers of the hypnotist as a potential benefactor.

As a transferential object in the form of a *parental surrogate,* the therapist plays his seventh role in the therapeutic drama. Once the idealization of the therapist crumbles to the dust of disappointment, the frustrations and furies of childhood, compounded out of significant early conditionings, may contaminate the relationship with the therapist (Gill and Brenman[6]). The distortion of the image of the therapist is often concealed by pleasantries, defenses, and facades; but dreams, fantasies, and associations may expose the undercurrent interpersonal climate. Unless the therapist is trained to detect and to deal with transferential symbols, resistance may soon block therapeutic progress. Hypnosis can expedite the release of transference in a remarkable way and lay open insidious roadblocks to memory recovery.

The eighth common role of the therapist is that of *educator.* Patients will obviously look up to the therapist for constructive guidance. They will seek counsel and direction to usher them out of the middle of their neurotic plight. But unfortunately they will block their own path with resistances—resistances to the development of a proper working relationship, to the understanding of the nature and source of their problems, to the use of the therapist's techniques, to the employment of reparative and restorative patterns, to the control of their own destiny. Dealing with these resistances is perhaps the most important task in moving a patient from dead center. Hypnosis not only serves an important function in detecting and exposing the myriad resistances to change, but it helps the patient to challenge and work them through.

When we consider the multiple roles that the therapist must play in psychotherapy, we come to the conclusion that the quality of his personality which will enable him to assume the varied roles demanded of him will be as important as his expertise. Hypnosis will not overcome deficiencies in the therapist that interfere with capacities to function in various therapeutic roles. The therapist will respond to the patient, not only as one who needs his help, but also as an individual onto whom he can project certain of his own needs and problems. These may run counter to the essential roles he must assume. We may anticipate varied strivings in the therapist, his reactions being influenced by the sex, status, age, attitudes, symptoms, and personality characteristics of the patient. Thus the same therapist may react sadistically toward a strong male patient, with pathological tenderness toward a weak passive male, with seductive feelings toward an attractive female, with violent disgust toward a drug addict, and with hopelessness toward a schizophrenic. The presence in the therapist of therapeutically destructive attitudes can be antagonistic to improvement with any kind of psychotherapy. The mere fact that he employs hypnosis will not make up for bankruptcy in any of his personality assets.

The basic requirements for good hypnotic therapy are no different from those for any kind of brief psychotherapy. The therapist must be able to perceive rapidly the underlying dynamics and immediate emotional needs, and to recognize what constructive defenses and other assets exist that will aid him in helping his patients respond positively to him and to his techniques.

The value of hypnosis is thus no greater than the proficiency of the practitioner who employs it. There are many professionals who do well with other techniques, but who refuse to use hypnosis because they are not able to employ it competently. Actually not all doctors make good surgeons, and not all therapists can become competent hypnotherapists. Some fail miserably when they attempt to practice the hypnotic method. Skill is an ingredient in any technique and hypnosis is no exception. What is important for each therapist to establish is the utility for him of hypnosis in his work. Does he feel comfortable in utilizing hypnosis? Does inducing a trance make him feel powerful, sadistic, or anxious? Does he sense a change in his feelings toward his hypnotized subject which differ from how he feels when the patient is in the waking state? Is he able to remain objective about the material produced by the patient? Can he apply the same dynamic criteria to the behavior responses of the patient in hypnosis, and to the patient's reactions to the trance experience posthypnotically, as he would to any other of the patient's reactions? Does hypnosis have a personal meaning for the therapist that makes him overvalue its effects? These questions can be answered only when the therapist applies his hypnotic technique to a variety of patients and carefully observes his own responses as well as those of his subjects. Where untoward feelings are mobilized in him, he may ask himself whether he can control these feelings in order to operate as objectively as possible. If he cannot, hypnosis is not a technique that is suitable for him.

One common defect is excessive passivity in the therapist. There is a tradition in training that dictates that one must be as inactive and noninterfering as possible. The presumption is that the patient must dictate the terms of his own destiny, as well as the pace he pursues in approaching a cure. The therapist must do nothing to interpose his own values on the patient since the patient must work these out for himself. Theoretically this sounds fine. The only problem is that the methods that derive from these precepts help very few patients. In most cases a structured and rational kind of activity guarantees the best results. A good therapist does not impose his standards on his patient; however, he has a responsibility to interfere with ideas and attitudes that are part of cherished value systems which the patient insists on retaining even though they are to his continued disadvantage.

What is vital also is that the therapist feel free to interrupt neurotic symptoms if necessary without worrying too much about whether or not he is doing something antitherapeutic. An unwholesome shibboleth in psychiatry is the belief that although symptoms may be temporarily ameliorated by suggestion, a cure cannot be achieved until the motive for recovery overwhelms the ends achieved by the illness, or until the dynamic psychological processes which mediate the disease are thoroughly understood by the patient himself. Remove a symptom and its return in the same or substitutive form will hang over the patient like the sword of Damocles. An illustrative but apocryphal story is that of a hiccuping applicant at an airline office who requested a ticket from an unusually attractive clerk. "Here you are," remarked the girl, "and you owe us an additional $150." "What! " exclaimed the man indignantly. "I paid for my ticket completely." He continued excitedly, "I don't owe you a cent more." "I know," smiled the clerk flirtatiously, "but you see, I cured your hiccups." Looking surprised the man replied, "You are absolutely right. Now what can you do for high blood pressure? "

There is still, in spite of overwhelming clinical evidence of its safety, controversy about symptom removal. In a few experimental situations that have been reported by several investigators, symptoms removed by direct command without any suggestion as to replacement have produced some substitute symptoms (Seitz[9,10]); however, the same kind of experiments done by other observers have not shown this result. In either case, the attitude and expectations of the operator may be somehow communicated to the patient, perhaps nonverbally. I have personally tried to bring on vicarious symptoms by forceful suggestions. At least with my techniques I have either successfully removed or ameliorated the symptoms without ill effect, or else the patient has refused to abandon them in spite of my best efforts. In the latter instance I presume the patients needed their symptoms to preserve their psychological balance. The goal of symptom relief is a legitimate one, for any disturbing symptomatology results in a pyramiding of tension which may cue off a variety of physical and emotional ailments not directly related to the original complaint. It follows that removal of an offensive symptom can restore the individual's sense of mastery rather than vitiate it, and restoration of emotional homeostasis may then result.

There is considerable evidence that supportive and palliative techniques may sometimes result not only in lasting relief from complaints, but also, in some cases, even in reconstructive character change (Wolberg[14]). These developments are not fortuitous. They follow the working through of conflict initiated by a constructive use of the therapeutic interpersonal relationship. What happens, it may be asked, if a patient insists upon retaining a certain symptom though he realizes it is neurotic and even self-damaging? I believe that it is within a patient's rights to retain a symptom if he really desires to do so. But when a patient comes to me with a crippling symptom, and tells me that he does not want to give his symptom up, I feel it to be an obligation to help him to reposition his sights. Many patients forced to see me by their physicians because of excess tension or improper life habits would like to get well without altering in the least the destructive patterns responsible for their troubles. Sometimes they will want me to force them to want to get well. Obviously this is impossible with hypnosis or with any other technique; however, I will try to educate them into recognizing for themselves their improper thinking processes that make them adhere to values and patterns that are hurtful to them. But in the long run they are the arbiters of their own destiny and eventually must make the choice between retaining strivings that make for illness and those that will promote health.

Another common question is why if a patient really wants to get well, he is sometimes unable, even when his motivation for recovery is strong, to overcome his neurosis in spite of our best skills as hypnotherapists. One deterrent to our therapeutic designs is the emergence of outmoded coping mechanisms that survive in almost pristine form, even though the paths toward which they are pressed serve destructive ends. Much as cultures retain folkways of primitive lineage that have no functional utility, so the human being repetitively and compulsively is committed to anachronistic means of attack, retreat, entrenchment, and other defenses. These we employed in defiance of reason as preferred modes of interpersonal operation. Flexibility to shifts in the environment is the keynote of adaptation; inflexibility cannot help but interfere with mental health.

What actually accounts for the peculiarly tenacious persistence of maladaptive and functionally useless patterns is difficult to say. Neither psychoanalytic theory nor learning theory nor any other theory has adequately explained them. One would expect that the absence of positive reinforcements would eventually extinguish certain traits particularly where they have created problems for the individual. But even though no rewards are apparent, some neurotic patterns persist to the mutual dismay of the victim and the professional person who proposes to help him.

It is in the therapy of such apparently nonresponsive patients that a dynamic approach can prove valuable above and beyond the benefits of symptom removal. One cannot discount the effectiveness of nondynamic behavioral approaches in the average individual. These often depreciate the delving into unconscious material and the disgorging of repressed and repudiated aspects of the psyche. But in many recalcitrant patients we find that a mere search for immediate environmental reinforcements of maladaptive behavior, and efforts to remove these or to substitute for them unpleasant consequences yields little for our efforts. Moreover, where the behavioral repertoire needs broadening and attempts are made to remove behavioral deficits by techniques which reward for proper responses, we are disappointed in the hoped-for shaping of healthy conduct.

Where a therapist has had some psychoanalytic training he may be able to expand his effectiveness by probing into the sources of conflict in his nonresponsive patients. It is not always essential to burrow into the depths of the unconscious with all the techniques that Freud has given us. The patient will usually reveal basic problems to us without effort by his defiant responses to our methods and to our personalities as we induce hypnosis and utilize the trance to pursue our therapeutic objectives. Resistance to hypnotherapy will reflect fundamental characterologic distortions and surviving childish needs and defenses which act as initiating foci for neurotic illness. In bringing the patient to an awareness of his resistances and manipulations, we are often enabled to break through the impediments that without challenge will surely cripple our best therapeutic tactics. The hypnotic experience becomes a biopsy of the existing pathology and ultimately a means to its resolution.

What may happen then is an insightful working through of neurotic patterns. Theoretically repressions are restored to keep certain pathogenic conflicts from awareness. A more harmonious balance occurs among the various components of the psychic apparatus. A sense of mastery permits the discarding of regressive defenses. Positive reinforcements are then imparted for productive behavior while neurotic behavior receives negative reinforcement.

Where resistances to verbalization, free association, and the remembering of dreams and early memories exist, hypnosis may lift these obstructions (Wolberg[15]). Hypnosis may light up archaic interfering transference and bring fundamental problems to the surface. It may also aid in the working-through process, particularly the conversion of insight into action by dealing directly with resistances to change.

It is difficult to see how the dimensions of transference and resistance which occur in one form or another in many patients even in the briefest hypnotic therapy can be managed without some knowledge of, and capacity to work within, a dynamically oriented framework. Furthermore, countertransference is so often mobilized in active approaches such as hypnosis that its understanding and control are mandatory to effective operation. Actually the understanding of psychoanalytic principles may enable us to follow more accurately a patient's progress and to detect resistance even where our goal is mere symptom relief. Such understanding may spell the difference between success and failure.

The notion that in the trance state we bypass resistances to deal exclusively with the unconscious (Freud[5]), only to have the conscious barriers restored with awakening, is another of the persistent misconceptions about hypnosis. Any experienced analyst is aware of the need to work with resistances rather than with the repudiated drives and conflicts that evade the resistances. The uncovering of repressed material may come about with the hypnotic induction or the use of certain hypnoanalytic techniques. This is insufficient in itself. What is required is that the patient be challenged to understand why it is difficult for him to countenance or to acknowledge this material to the waking state. Pointed questions and injunctions to work on his resistances, and to accept, reject, or modify the material that has been revealed while pondering its implications, may register their effects on the patient's ego. The changes wrought will be manifest in the patient's dreams—for instance, in less distorted symbolism and conscious associations. "Spontaneous" insights may then emerge.

We must overemphasize the need for insight in all cases. In my experience, and that of many of my colleagues, the overcoming of an established neurotic pattern can occur without the subjective appearance of insight. What often happens is that insight *follows* upon the resolution of a problem, rather than precedes it. For example, a frigid woman who experiences her first orgasm may be rewarded with a flood of insights into why she feared yielding control, which will help her to face intercourse with expectations of enjoyment rather than frustration.

This is not to minimize the impact of true understanding of the repetitive and compulsive nature of contemporary neurotic behavior, and its origins in early life experience with significant authority figures. This type of insight may act as a liberating force from the primary and secondary gains of the neurosis. It upsets the balance between the repressed and repressing elements. It fosters a desire to test the reality of one's attitudes and values. It gives the person an opportunity to challenge the very philosophies that govern his life. But insight alone is not enough to arrest the neurotic process and to promote new and constructive ways of handling reality. Instead, insight may produce not change but an accentuation of anxiety, since it defies the individual to approach life on different terms. He is perhaps for the first time outraged at his customary defensive tactics. He may then throw up a smoke screen of resistance and retreat into old defensive patterns. Therapy may grind to a halt induced by intolerable fantasies associated with action.

It is at this point that the dynamic therapist can utilize the precepts of those who are dedicated to symptom-oriented therapy, as are the behavior theorists. He can encourage his patients, once they have acquired "insight," to expose themselves actively to situations which will ablate unhealthful and reinforce constructive behavior. Hypnosis can be singularly effective in promoting such an exposure (Spiegel,[12] Moss[7]). There is much in the methods of both behavior therapists and those who are psychoanalytically oriented for mutual study and blending if they retain experimental open-mindness and discard their distrust of each other.

We may challenge another questionable traditional precept: the idea that hypnosis is unsuited for certain vulnerable patients: for instance, borderline cases who are notoriously unstable and who are likely to shift over into a psychotic phase at the least sign of stress. In my experience I have found hypnosis particularly suited to the treatment of many borderline patients. By promoting relaxation, it can have a calming effect on the individual. I believe that it may, in the existing protective atmosphere of a relationship with a projected idealized supportive, nonpunitive authority figure, be singularly reassuring. The interested, nonthreatening encouraging manner of the operator, with absence of hostile and seductive maneuvers, may be most supportively rewarding. This is not to say that the patient will not respond with misinterpretation and unstable behavior irrespective of how gently he is appraoched. But a proper bearing on the part of the operator reduces such incidents and may be therapeutically rewarding.

Obviously one must expect in some borderline patients during hypnosis a greater degree of emotionally disturbed reactions than in more stable patients. These reactions may spontaneously erupt irrespective of the approach or behavior of the operator. They are easily provoked by overt aggressive activities, or probing. They are most frequently mobilized by psychotherapeutic techniques that challenge defenses and resistances, or that deal with preconscious or unconscious trends and impulses. They are less frequently present when during hypnosis suggestions are confined to tension alleviation or pain reduction. They are reduced by a reassuring and supportive attitude on the part of the operator.

There is, therefore, no reason why hypnosis should not be used in borderline and even psychotic patients. But where an operator finds that he is excessively upset by occasional disturbed reactions, or is unable to control them, or observes that he stimulates more than occasional explosiveness in such patients, he may prudently avoid hypnosis. This is not to say that in the waking state he may not be confronted with similar upsetting reactions in his sicker cases, particularly where his techniques or the relationship is interpreted as threatening. However, it may be that his own unconscious manipulations and aggressive or seductive tendencies may not reveal themselves so easily in his tactics without hypnosis.

There is no way of predicting in advance the exact influence that hypnosis may have on any patient or his problems, since each individual will respond uniquely to the techniques in line with the special meanings they have for him. The mental set with which he approaches hypnosis, his motivations to be helped, the depth and quality of his resistances, his conception of the therapist and the image he conjures up of him, the skill of the therapist, the kinds of interventions administered, the management of the patient's doubts and oppositional tendencies, and the nature of the patient's transference and therapist's countertransference will all enter into the responsive Gestalt.

Potentially hypnosis may catalyze every aspect of the therapeutic process. Whether or not the therapist will want to employ it will depend largely on how much confidence he has in hypnosis and how well he works with hypnotic techniques. I believe that every therapist owes it to himself to experiment with hypnosis as an adjunct to his customary psychotherapeutic methods, for if he gives himself the proper opportunity, he may as a consequence be able greatly to enhance his effectiveness as a psychotherapist. The least that can happen is that he will learn a great deal more about the workings of the human mind than he knew before in his prehypnotic days. And this in itself can be a cherished blessing.

REFERENCES

1. Conn, J. H.: The Psychodynamics of Recovery Under Hypnosis. Int. J. Clin. Exp. Hypn. 8:3-15, 1960.
2. Dorcus, R. M.: The Influence of Hypnosis on Learning and Habit Modifying. In: Dorcus, R. M. (Ed.), Hypnosis and Its Therapeutic Applications. New York, McGraw-Hill Book Co., Inc., 1956.
3. Dreikurs, R.: The Interpersonal Relationship in Hypnosis. Psychiatry 25:219-226, 1962.
4. Frank, J.: Persuasion and Healing: A Comparative Study of Psychotherapy. Baltimore, Johns Hopkins Press, 1961.
5. Freud, A.: The Ego and the Mechanisms of Defense. New York, International Universities Press, 1946.
6. Gill, M. M., and Brenman, M.: The Metapsychology of Regression and Hypnosis. In: Gordon, J. E. (Ed.), Handbook of Clinical and Experimental Hypnosis. New York, The Macmillan Company, 1967, pp. 281-318.
7. Moss, C. S.: Brief Crisis-Oriented Hypnotherapy. In: Gordon, J. E. (Ed.), Handbook of Clinical and Experimental Hypnosis. New York, The Macmillan Company, 1967.
8. Orne, M. T.: Implications for Psychotherapy Derived from Current Research on the Nature of Hypnosis. Amer. J. Psychiat. 118:1097-1103, 1962.
9. Seitz, P. F.: Symbolism and Organ Choice in Conversion Reactions: An Experimental Approach. Psychosom. Med. 13:255-259, 1951.
10. Seitz, P. F.: Experiments in the Substitution of Symptoms by Hypnosis. II. Psychosom. Med. 14:405-424, 1953.
11. Shapiro, A. K.: Attitudes Toward the Use of Placebos in Treatment. J. Nerv. Ment. Dis. 130:200-211, 1960.
12. Spiegel, H.: Hypnotic Intervention as an Adjunct for Rapid Clinical Relief. Int. J. Clin. Exp. Hypn. 10:23-29, 1963.
13. Weitzenhoffer, A. M., and Sjoberg, B. M.: Suggestibility with and Without "Induction of Hypnosis." J. Nerv. Ment. Dis. 132:204-220, 1961.
14. Wolberg, L. R.: The Technic of Short-Term Psychotherapy. In: Wolberg, L. R. (Ed.), Short-Term Psychotherapy. New York, Grune & Stratton, Inc., 1965, pp. 127-200.
15. Wolberg, L. R.: Hypnoanalysis. In: Wolman, B. B. (Ed.), Psychoanalytic Techniques. New York, Basic Books, Inc., 1967, pp. 533-559.

Reality Therapy

by William Glasser, M.D., and Leonard M. Zunin, M.D.

Reality therapy is based upon the premise that all people in all cultures possess from birth to death a need for an identity; that no other person thinks, looks, acts, and talks exactly as each individual does. Reality therapy differs from psychoanalysis, from operant conditioning, or from some of the newer therapeutic ideas in that it is applied not only to the problems of irresponsibility and incompetence, but also to the modes of daily living.

Formation of a success or failure identity becomes most obvious at age 6, when the child enters the first grade and is first challenged to develop intellectual, verbal, and social skills which determine if he will be a successful or unsuccessful person and associate with others accordingly. Individuals who identify with failure either *deny* reality or *ignore* it. What is traditionally called mental illness are the various methods by which an individual avoids reality.

The Basic Principles of Reality Therapy

Basic to reality therapy is the concept of involvement, which is necessary to motivate a person toward success. The following are ways in which the therapist becomes responsibly involved with the person he is trying to help and guides him toward working for a success identity.

Principle I: Personal

The therapist must communicate that he cares, that he is warm and friendly. Aloofness and cool detachment are not therapeutic. Understanding and realistic concern are the cornerstones of effective treatment. The use of personal pronouns by both the therapist and the patient such as *I* and *me* and *you,* rather than *it* or *one does* or *out there* or *they,* facilitates involvement.

Being personal also means that the therapist is willing, if indicated and appropriate, to discuss his own experiences and to have his values challenged and discussed. He demonstrates that he acts in a responsible manner and admits that he is far from being perfect or free of concerns. The therapist conveys to the individual, usually nonverbally, his sincere belief that the patient has the ability to be happier and do better, and that he is capable of functioning in a more responsible, effective, and self-fulfilling manner. In fact, if the therapist does not believe this about the patient, he is doing the patient a disservice by continuing to engage him in a treatment situation.

It is not possible for a therapist who leads a responsible life of his own to become deeply involved in friendships with everyone who comes to him for help except within the context of the office. The therapist has to be honest about this and explain it to the patient, rather than imply promises which he cannot fulfill. The warmth, the concern, the involvement in the therapeutic relationship, is what is essential, rather than the content of the verbal exchange. This means that anything is open for discussion; if the individual is talking about subjects other than his own misery or problems, this is not seen as resistance but rather as something worthwhile and of interest to both the therapist and the patient.

Principle II: Focus on Behavior Rather Than Feelings

There is a basic fallacy in the notion "When I feel better, I will do more;" when people do more, they feel better. It is far easier to enter this cycle at the "doing" rather than the "feeling" point.

For example, if an individual comes to the office and states, "I feel miserable and depressed," rather than one of the traditional answers such as silence or "Tell me more about it," or "Have you had any suicidal thoughts? " or "Have you ever felt this depressed at any other time in your life? " the reality therapist might respond by saying, "Is it possible that what you are doing is depressing you? " When patients begin to outline what they are doing and what they have done over the last few days, it often becomes apparent that any normal, average human being would also be depressed with similar conduct. The therapist might then ask the patient why he was not more depressed—a provocative question for most individuals seeking help. When they begin, with the help of the therapist, to outline the various modes of conduct that support them emotionally and prevent their becoming ever further depressed, we assist them in becoming aware of their own inner strengths, potentials, and attributes.

This second principle is poignantly illustrated in intimate love relationships. Unless two individuals enjoy each other as human beings, the feelings of love and warmth and closeness begin to fade. Only by sharing behavior, whether sexually or in constructive and creative enjoyment, can the relationship be sustained and grow.

Principle III: Focus on the Present

Reality therapy is based upon a conviction that whatever we are today is the sum total of everything that has happened in our lives; however, all that can be changed is the immediate present and the future. When the past is discussed, incidents are never left as entities in and of themselves but are always related to current behavior. For example, if a person described a crisis experience that occurred several years ago, the therapist will ask him what he learned from it, and how it is related to his present behavior and attempts to succeed in life. In contrast to traditional psychotherapeutic approaches, which emphasize past traumatic encounters, failures, and difficulties, (1) we discuss strengthening and character-building experiences that occurred in the individual's past and relate them to current attempts to succeed, (2) we explore constructive alternatives that the individual might have taken at the time, and (3) we discuss especially what he did do that assisted him in avoiding greater difficulty.

Contrary to this principle, case histories in the traditional format, whether by probation officers, psychiatrists, psychologists, or social workers, sometimes concentrate on failures, shortcoming, traumas, and problems with which the person has had to cope, whereas a person's successes and hidden potentials are sadly neglected.

Principle IV: Value Judgments

Every patient must make a value judgment as to what he is doing to contribute to his own failure before he can be helped to change. Part of emotional health is a willingness to work within the framework of society. However, the therapist should not impose his own social judgments on the patient, since this would relieve the patient of the responsibility for his own behavior.

Principle V: Planning and Commitment

One of the continual problems in therapy, as well as in all aspects of life, is that, once a good plan is made, we must develop the strength and the responsibility to carry it through. A significant portion of therapy involves making plans that are realistic. It is far better to err on the side of programs that are simple and easily implemented, than those that are complex and stand a greater risk of failure. Patients gain a success identity only through successes and not through failures.

An important advantage is to put the plan in writing, particularly in the form of a contract betwee n patient and therapist. The differential weight that is attached to the written versus the spoken word was long ago utilized by the legal profession, and the reality therapist may find this an exceedingly useful device.

Principle VI: Evasions

Plans may fail, but it is the obligation of the reality therapist to make clear to the patient that no excuses are acceptable. Far more therapeutic benefit is gained from working with the patient on redeveloping the plan than in discussing the reasons for the plan's failure. The therapist should not deprecate the patient for failing, but the joint task is to make a new plan or to modify the old one.

Principle VII: Eliminate Punishment

Punishment works most poorly on individuals with a failure identity. Therefore, we avoid ridicule, sarcasm, or hostile statements such as "You just don't have what it takes."

Punishment is different from the natural consequences of failure. To the extent that the reality therapist is able to eliminate punishment and not accept excuses for failure, to help the patient substitute constructive value judgments and make plans accordingly, and then help him to make a commitment to follow through, the therapist is assisting his patient to achieve success.

Transference, as described in other therapeutic approaches, occurs not only in the therapeutic experience but in the experiences of everyday life. Rather than attempt to enhance this phenomenon and then "analyze" it, the reality therapist attempts to decrease attendant distortions. If the patient relates to the reality therapist by saying, "You remind me of my father," the reality therapist may say, "I am not your father, but I would be interested in knowing what you see in us as similar." The therapist thus attempts in every way possible to present himself as a genuine, concerned person, helping the patient to understand and deal with reality.

Practical Pastoral Counseling*

by Calvert Stein, M.D.

The Pastoral Mystique

Pastors outnumber psychiatrists by about 35 to 1, and psychologists by about 15 to 1. Although no longer the awesome witch doctor and traditional medicine man of his tribe, the pastor is frequently the first port of call in times of trouble. Pastors often make heroic efforts to bridge the generation gap and to facilitate expression of contemporary concern in the search for a meaning to life.

Traditional tools of the pastoral calling still include an ecclesiastic mantle, brief prayer, appropriate scriptural quotation or incantation representing a higher authority, and an attentive ear. These procedures promote a natural hypnotic receptivity per se, even without the bowed head and priestly touch. They are also inherent in the spiritual aura which the pastor carries with him to homes, meetings, and hospitals.

Regardless of setting, however, the daily observance of simple ritual, religious symbols, and sacred music serve as excellent tranquilizers for the anxious and troubled believer, but agnostics and atheists are not entirely immune.

As with ancient high priests the clerical garb may be scant defense against staunch defenders of tradition. Consequently the modern pastor risks much when he attempts radical departures from prescribed ritual by bringing into a previously conservative house of worship such changes as vernacular prayer books, rock and roll, folk masses, "sensitivity" groups, and other "heretical" abominations. Emotional turmoil can be minimized when changes are made gradually.

When to Consult or Refer

Self-Referral. Like miracle workers of old the pastor usually recognizes the intimate relations between mind and body—the psychosomatic pain, the flush, flutter, tremor, dry mouth, and other tensions (cf. *pulpit jitters;* Job 17:1, 19:14). He also respects the efficacy of adjunctive faith healing as well as the restraining potency of an implied "hex" via spiritual disapproval. Nevertheless,

---

*Some of the material in this chapter appeared in somewhat different form in *Practical Pastoral Counseling,* by Calvert Stein, Springfield, Ill., Charles C Thomas, 1970. Courtesy of the publisher.

he too must learn to deal with personal pressures including temptation, seduction, betrayal, disillusionment, guilt, and self-reproach from his own mistakes—especially failure to deal with transference and countertransference.[6] He must also "play it cool" with competitive colleagues and obstreperous lay associates who frequently reject what they actually need.

Recognition of Emotional Depression. The patient or client with morbid and sometimes unrecognized emotional depression often has physical complaints which are resistive to all therapy except temporarily to euphoric drugs or alcohol. He makes many promises but few friends and cannot keep them because he is usually dull company except when he can have "just one or two" drinks. As Al-Anon repeatedly reminds the spouses, alcoholics are experts at the confidence game, but physical as well as moral degradation are close behind, and the treatment is neither short nor simple.[1,2] Families, employers, or "friends" who cover up for addicts are doing them no favors. The addiction not only serves as a camouflage for self-destruction—it also offers a quasi alibi for involving and endangering others.

Taking unnecessary risks, ignoring customary safety precautions, habitual overwork, habitual clowning, and giving away valuable personal belongings may be the first clues to underlying depression. Too many emergency wards still fail to insist on psychiatric care.

Another risk is the borderline would-be suicide who will not give his name or extracts a promise not to tell anyone or appeals to the counselor's vanity: "You're the only one I can trust." Such a precarious client needs strength, not honor or sentiment. Calling the police may be distasteful and embarrassing yet easier to face than guilty negligence and irreversible death.

Sharing Responsibility. In general, what is true for the alcoholic, drug user, and suicidal client also applies to the homosexual, habitual gambler, criminal, shoplifter, and recidivist juvenile delinquent. Their misconduct represents both rebellion and a thinly veiled cry for help.

Parents who physically abuse their children need sterner correction than a pastor can usually supervise, but the field is still wide open for his constructive influence. Too much negligence, indulgence, and leniency not only on the part of parents but also by judges and society is largely responsible for each community's having the kind of morality and safety which it deserves.

Miscellaneous Challengers. The isolate or loner is an expert at avoiding commitments. The harder one tries to help him, the more he resists.

The chronic disrespecter of other people's rights or privacy appeals to sympathy, expects extra privileges, and pays little attention to what others say or think. Giving him "enough rope" may hang the project as well as himself. This is especially true of the "eager beaver" helper who wants to be in on everything, tries to hog the credit, but lets others carry the ball and do the work.*

Sociopathic dropouts make their own rules yet follow them only when convenient. For these misanthropes argument and reason are usually futile. In a captive audience, as in an institutional setting, they have been known to respond to group confrontation by their peers as well as renewed religious pressure. However, hard-core homosexuals, alcoholics, and drug addicts are usually the result of long-standing emotional deprivation and warping. Consequently, preventive treatment requires early detection, complete abstinence, and intensive long-term reconstruction by devoted experts.

Common Denominators in Counseling and Psychotherapy

Pastoral counseling arose from the universal demand for protection from the great unknown, for an explanation of the mysteries of birth, puberty, sickness, death, floods, and other disasters, and for control of the unseen spirits that affected man's destiny. ". . . for with authority commandeth he even the unclean spirits, and they do obey him" (Mark 1:27).

Faith healing is based on the universal power of positive suggestion in a group of two or more—patient, clergyman, and God. Suggestibility and receptivity are enhanced by the priestly touch, concentrated attention, exclusion of extraneous stimuli, heightened expectation of gratifying results, and the willingness to make some personal sacrifice. These are also the phenomena of the hypnotherapeutic trance state. Assuredly no psychedelic drug could be expected to accomplish more.

Major procedures in counseling, faith healing, and psychotherapy are also universal, regardless of varying "new" doctrines and tongue-twisting terminology. They can be recognized as familiar principles of worship: meditation, ventilation of grievances, emotional release or abreaction of tension from anxiety, cleansing via confession and ritual, atonement via sacrifice, payment, or penance, and reformation of behavior.

These psychotherapeutic procedures serve the faithful followers by affording favorable opportunities to "cool it" and to learn how to "hang loose" when they are "uptight." They can be as productive over the telephone or at the bedside as in the sanctuary—especially with the additional bonus of the benediction.

The benediction or summing up should also review such issues as: What has been accomplished thus far? What are the long-range objectives? What must be tackled immediately? What liabilities must be overcome? And what strengthening assets make the task less difficult than it had appeared at first? For the

---

*A second reading of the parable of the prodigal son may help to refocus attention on the underlying injustice of an overindulgent father toward a conscientious and hard-working brother (Luke 15:11-32).

self-styled atheist one may suggest approval from some appropriate VIP whether living or dead as a substitute for divine approval. In everyone's life some mortal had to care.

Productive Techniques in Personal Counseling

Initial Contact. When on call the pastoral counselor should be available at all times yet avoid making commitments he cannot keep. In the initial summons he should note omissions, repetitions, contradictions, gross errors, and freudian slips; he should make a house visit if indicated or suggest another telephone or office conference soon, and perhaps a letter meanwhile. The caller may be completely in the wrong, yet the pastor usually does better with a soft answer. He can always be sorry for something; e.g., "I'm sorry you feel this way" or "I'm sorry so few people agree with you, but I'm glad you're thinking the problem through" or "I appreciate your calling to express your views."

Like the country doctor of old the pastor is always on call. Nevertheless, to protect his health and privacy, he must also learn how to say "no" diplomatically; e.g., "I have an emergency call at the hospital but I can make time for you later in the day" or "Drop in for a chat right after the next service" or "Please write me a letter and I'll certainly make the time to read it. Meanwhile, shall we pray together...?" or "Let's bring it up at tomorrow's open conference" or "Several others have had a similar problem and are eager for a group discussion. We meet right after vespers; and you don't have to talk about yourself if you don't want to.... I'm sure you'll feel lots better.... I'll be looking for you; and thank you very much for calling."

When brief services are held regularly several times each day, they operate as a continuing therapeutic group experience. A familiar example of this among orthodox and conservative Jews is the breakfast minyan at which 10 or more bereaved mourners gather for daily kaddish memorial prayers followed by fellowship and food which they prepare themselves.

Useful relaxing procedures while talking in the pastor's study include such "busy work" as knitting, doodling, finger painting, and clay modeling. They serve as constructive nonverbal outlets like caressing a rosary. They displace conscious attention and also afford some feelings of accomplishment as well as security.

Maintaining a strong image by the counselor requires cultivation of appropriate diction and meticulous attention to personal cleanliness—especially shoes, nails, and breath. Levity, off-color stories, inappropriate diction, and personal anecdotes are inappropriate. The counselor should not confide similar mistakes or doubts of his own. When a personal anecdote seems indicated, it can be told in the third person as though it had happened to a friend or acquaintance.

Clay Modeling. From an assortment of small plastic jars of modeling clay on the counselor's desk, the client is invited to select a sample. His choice of color usually harmonizes with tie, shirt, blouse, or dress and usually reflects the mood of the day. "While we are talking just let your hands do whatever they feel like doing with the clay." A perfectionist frequently models a sphere or "perfect world." A hostile client may refuse yet make a crude baseball which he would obviously like to throw at someone. The counselor may then invite him to punch a pillow held by the counselor, or bang down on a chair or sofa, or play a game of darts on the board on which any VIP or s.o.b. may be projected. When a client models a flower (the sex organ of plants), he may be preoccupied with spiritual love for a departed soul; however, when a hangman's noose or a lethal weapon is fashioned, confrontation and consultation are usually in order. Clients will often hastily destroy their creations if the models are too obviously associated with an embarrassing conflict. Nests, eggs, and fruit bowls suggest home and family. Vague or impressionistic creations usually conceal the sculptor's hidden message. Snapshots can be taken of the production and the subject reviewed at a later conference.

Role playing is a simple adaptation of an old counseling procedure: "Well, what would you do in my place? " It is an effective game of make-believe. The counselor says, "All right. Now you know this person who's been upsetting you. Let's pretend you are that person. You try to mimic him so I'll have a fairly clear idea of what he's like. I know you, and I'll try to think, talk, and act as you might do."

When the client is unable to assume another's role or to remain in that role, a personal hang-up is obviously indicated. The counselor then relieves the tension or embarrassment by changing the subject or reversing roles or even playing both roles. Role playing stops when it has accomplished its objective or is no longer productive. Frequently no words are needed at all. A spontaneous gesture, whether hostile, friendly, or indifferent, may convey one's feelings more eloquently.

Roles are reversed whenever clarification is needed. After a few starts the client may exclaim, "Oh, but she wouldn't *say* that" or "It wouldn't happen that way." The counselor then invites role reversal so the client can show just what "she" would have said or done. Insights usually develops rapidly but the experienced counselor does not have to confront the client or spell it out every time. It is usually enough to say, "How do you feel now? "

When role playing and role reversal are used in groups, others are invited to express how they feel. Common denominators are usually reported in the form of childhood frustrations, injustices, unexpressed grievances, and inability to deal with people who habitually impose. Presently, additional psychodramas with rehearsal for dreaded future interviews are enacted among smaller subgroups in various parts of the room. The leader merely invites the members to "rap" or chat with anyone they like while he either leaves the room or makes the rounds and visits with each group as auditor or participant after asking the group's permission.

Additional Rewarding Group Procedures

Warm-up techniques include music, songs, hymns, a processional march, dancing, games, projects, busy work, and other community center routines. Natural dominance will emerge from leaderless groups left to themselves, but the dominance is not necessarily constructive—even well-meaning catalyzers often need controls.

The simulated hot line introduces hypothetical situations for "safe" confrontation. Several volunteers man a simulated 24-hour telephone answering service for "troubled callers." The pastor may act as observer or director. The "caller" may refuse to reveal his name or telephone number but the "panelist" may also fail to make adequate contact and consequently loses his chance to help. Statements such as the following can be productive: "Thank you very much for calling. You may call me John, and I'd like you to choose some name by which I can call you. It doesn't have to be your real name. I also want you to know that I will not hang up on you but you do know that telephone disconnections sometimes happen; so if you'll let me have the number I could call you right back. You'd rather not? Okay. I just wanted you to know. Now, how can I help you? "

A "caller" may choose to report some crisis such as a "trip" with LSD or may threaten suicide or may describe some domestic scene. Personal identifications and analysis should be avoided. "How do the rest of you feel? " is a safe yet provocative question which offers the leader an opportunity to suggest, "Well then, suppose you reverse roles and let's see how it might go. Pretend that you (on the panel) really have this problem. Now change places with the 'caller' and show us what you would want someone to do about it? "

Management of Aggression

Verbal. A tense person is invited to think of a poem, song, or story, or to select someone from the group to take the role of an annoying person in his life (teacher, employer, member of family, a former buddy, or even the pastor himself) and to tell him or her off as a blankety-blank so-and-so, using whatever language he deems proper. Groups do not shock easily, and verbal retaliation with choice diction often releases unsuspected hostility or provokes unexpected laughter. Insight into identity of the real culprit often develops quickly.

A simple verbal warm-up procedure for any size group is to pair off the participants, who then choose a family or members of a team or make up a skit. One may say to the other, "There's something about you that I don't understand," or "Sometimes I think you don't like me," or "You bug me the wrong way," or some such remark. In short order each partner recognizes the need for further communication, and since it's a make-believe structured situation, they are usually able to accept and deal with the confrontation without too many defensive reactions.

Nonverbal. Members of the group pair off and choose a cast for a pantomime or charade. Or, facing each other, they lock hands and take turns trying to push each other around the room. Hand or "Indian" wrestling serves a similar purpose. A time limit of 5 to 10 seconds serves as a safety precaution. Or someone who feels left out can try to break into a circle of people who lock arms and try to exclude him. Similarly a timid person may be placed within a circle of his peers from which he is invited to try to break out. The rules should be clear: trickery or feints may be in, but foul play is out. When a member of a minority group succeeds on his own initiative, group approval usually appears spontaneously—even when someone in the circle lends a little help.

An excellent boost for morale results when eight volunteers (three on each side and one at head and feet) gently lift and then rock a prone isolate who has had a rough time and needs a little TLC: tender, loving care. Just sitting or reclining on a carpeted floor usually facilitates relaxation and simplifies the warm-up.[3]

Projective techniques are "make-believe" games in which everyone is invited to participate. As with a parable from scripture each auditor can identify as much as he chooses. A suggested verbalization using soothing tones follows: "Fix your gaze on some spot on the ceiling or wall. Keep watching it until your eyes get too heavy to stay open. Meanwhile let your breathing slow down, relax your body, make yourself very comfortable, and pretend to go sound asleep. Now the moment your eyes close I'd like you to imagine yourselves at a very special party. You've just won a door prize—something special and wonderful. You do not have to reveal the nature of your prize. However, when the party's over, just come back here, alert yourselves, and feel free to share with us as much as you are willing for us to know." [8]

For marriage counseling, any of the above procedures may prove effective. In addition, a study of the client's scrapbook, graduation and wedding pictures, reports on courtship, in-laws, honeymoon, work, eating, and other personal habits usually reveals the real culprit in the form of uncut apron strings and futile attempts to please or rebel against too many former competitors or VIPs. Be sure to ask who was *not* at the graduation, wedding, or other special event, and *why*.

Finally, the pastoral counselor is a patient teacher and a neutral referee—not a judge, jury, or partisan. The responsibility for accepting counseling and initiating change belongs with the individual client, who should be required to make his own appointments and commitments. You yourself are a VIP. Your own reputation for wisdom and firmness with finesse is being tested repeatedly; so do not hesitate to seek expert counseling when indicated. The world's best specialists for any problem are no further away than your own telephone.

For the dying patient one should provide truthful but compassionate reassurance, encouragement to sound off, and periodic suggestions to remember happier times. A gentle reminder of some of the wonderful "mystery trips" one used to take with a trusted adult serves as a positive influence to neutralize pessimism concerning the "last mile."

REFERENCES

1. Masserman, J. H.: Neurosis and Alcohol. In: Principles of Dynamic Psychiatry. Philadelphia, W. B. Saunders Company, 1946, pp. 210-215.
2. Masserman, J. H.: Causes and Dynamics of Alcoholism (#114). Pfizer Medical Film Library, New York, N.Y.
3. Schutz, E. C.: Joy. New York, Grove Press, Inc., 1969.
4. Stein, C.: Practical Psychotherapy in Nonpsychiatric Specialties. Springfield, Ill., Charles C Thomas, Publisher, 1969.
5. Stein, C.: Practical Family and Marriage Counseling. Springfield, Ill., Charles C Thomas, Publisher, 1970.
6. Stein, C.: Trance, Transference and Countertransference in the Resistive Patient. Amer. J. Clin. Hypn. 12:213-221 (April), 1970.
7. Stein, C.: Practical Pastoral Counseling. Springfield, Ill., Charles C Thomas, Publisher, 1970.
8. Stein, C.: Hypnotic Projection in Brief Psychotherapy. Amer. J. Clin. Hypn. pp. 143-155, 1970.
9. Stein, C.: Sex in the Bible. Unpublished data.

PART III

PSYCHOPHARMACOLOGY AND PHYSICAL MODALITIES

Pharmacotherapy of Tension and Anxiety

by Heinz E. Lehmann, M.D., and Thomas A. Ban, M.D.

Definition of Minor Tranquilizers

The word tranquilizer first appeared in the literature around 1822, used by DeQuincey, the author of *Confessions of an Opium Eater.* Thomas Hardy also used the term in the 1890s but after that the word practically disappeared from the language.[1] In the early 1950s it made a spectacular comeback, when the first effective drugs in the treatment of psychotic symptoms were discovered, i.e., chlorpromazine and reserpine.[2-4] It also happened that both these first two antipsychotic drugs produced drowsiness. They were therefore, somewhat hastily, labeled tranquilizers in order to distinguish them from other sedative and hypnotic drugs which produced drowsiness but which were ineffective against psychotic symptoms and which did not produce extrapyramidal manifestations. Within a short time a great number of drugs effective against psychosis and capable of inducing extrapyramidal signs were developed.[5] These also were called tranquilizers, along with new drugs which otherwise might or might not have fallen into the older classification of sedatives. So, in an attempt to prevent utter confusion, a distinction was made between "major" and "minor" tranquilizers—the major tranquilizers referring to the antipsychotics or neuroleptics and the *minor tranquilizers* referring to the antianxiety drugs which do not have any antipsychotic or neuroleptic effects.[6]

More recently the term anxiolytic sedatives has been proposed by the World Health Organization Committee[7] to cover any drugs which previously had been referred to as *minor tranquilizers.* The WHO defined anxiolytic sedatives as substances which reduce pathological anxiety, tension, and agitation without therapeutic effects on cognitive or perceptual processes. The qualification

70

"anxiolytic" was added to the old term sedative in order to indicate clearly that the focus of the classification was on the anxiety-reducing properties of these drugs. Hypnotics, sedatives, and minor tranquilizers were all grouped together as anxiolytic sedatives because the Committee agreed that there was insufficient evidence of a true pharmacological difference between them. All hypnotics—primarily sleep-inducing drugs—can be used effectively as anxiety-reducing sedatives when given in small enough doses, and all the drugs which are primarily and traditionally used for the treatment of anxiety and tension states—minor tranquilizers—induce drowsiness and sleep when given in sufficiently high doses.

Pharmacological Control of Anxiety

The history of the pharmacological control of anxiety, psychomotor restlessness, and insomnia can be separated into three periods: the first from the introduction of general anesthesia, which came into general use around 1850 (and subsequently of old-time sedatives), until the development of the first clinically used barbiturate in 1903; the second from the discovery of the barbiturates to the discovery of minor tranquilizers in the 1950s; and the third from that time until today's anxiolytic sedatives.

Minor Tranquilizers

There are three major groups of minor tranquilizers: propanediols, diphenyl-methanes, and benzodiazepines.

Propanediols. In the course of studies with phenylglycerol ethers in the 1940s—to develop compounds with antibacterial effects—Berger[8] found that some of the drugs produced flaccid paralysis of the voluntary skeletal muscles. Furthermore the phenylglycerol ether mephenesin exerted a quieting effect which was described as tranquilization in the first publication reporting on its pharmacological action.[9] It was of particular interest when it was shown that mephenesin could allay anxiety without clouding consciousness.[10,11] The rapid oxidation of mephenesin, however, seemed to be a clinical handicap, and attempts were made to produce a compound with longer duration of action. Various substitutions and esterifications of mephenesin finally resulted in meprobamate, a compound with a longer duration of action and a wider margin of safety. Among the propanediol derivatives which have found clinical application are ethinamate, primarily prescribed as a sleep-inducing agent, phenaglycodol, a daytime sedative, emylcamate, a substance with muscle-relaxing and tension-relieving properties, and tybamate, which has recently been introduced as an antianxiety drug.[12]

Both meprobamate and tybamate—the two most extensively employed propanediol preparations in the treatment of anxiety—are readily absorbed from the gastrointestinal tract. Meprobamate reaches its peak plasma levels 2 hours after ingestion and tybamate in less than 2 hours. This is followed by a steady decline in blood concentration. The half-life of meprobamate in the organism is 11 hours, whereas the half-life of tybamate is only 3 hours. Interestingly, physical dependence on tybamate has not been reported. Shelton and Hollister[13] attribute the absence of dependence and withdrawal reactions to the unusually short half-life of tybamate, which is only a third or a fourth of that of meprobamate.

Diphenylmethanes. Of the four minor tranquilizers in this category—benactyzine, captodiamine, hydroxyzine, and phenyltoloxamine—only one, hydroxyzine, is widely used in the treatment of anxiety. According to Lehmann,[14] an ideal anxiolytic should produce enough side effects to keep it from becoming habit forming ("to keep it a treatment rather than a treat"), but not so many as to reduce the patient's willingness to take it as prescribed. A recent study conducted by Silver et al.[15] suggests that hydroxyzine may approach these criteria.

Benzodiazepines. The benzodiazepines were derived from compounds known in the literature as 3,1,4-benzoxadiazepines. Since the discovery of chlordiazepoxide a large number of 1,4-benzodiazepines have been synthesized, studied pharmacologically, and investigated clinically. Among the benzodiazepine derivatives which have found clinical application are nitrazepam and flurazepam, primarily prescribed as sleep-inducing agents, and diazepam, oxazepam, medazepam, chlorazepate, and prazepam—all antianxiety drugs.

Other Anxiolytic Sedatives

There are several other relatively new groups of anxiolytic sedative drugs, e.g., carbinols, piperidinediones, quinazolones. Most recently doxepin, a dibenzoxepin derivative, was shown to have antianxiety effects. In a number of clinical studies doxepin was found to be at least as effective as an anxiolytic as some of the frequently employed minor tranquilizers, e.g., chlordiazepoxide, meprobamate, hydroxyzine, and phenobarbital. No case of dependency on doxepin has been reported to date.[16,17]

Are Minor Tranquilizers Effective?

In contrast to neuroleptics, the demonstration that minor tranquilizers have a therapeutic action encountered considerable difficulties. In two consecutive United States Veterans Administration (VA) studies, for example, no evidence could be found that the addition of an active drug has a superior therapeutic effect to an inactive placebo in the treatment of anxious patients.[18-20] On the other hand, the Philadelphia group, Rickels and his collaborators,[21] were able to demonstrate the superiority of minor tranquilizers—barbiturates, meprobamate, chlordiazepoxide, diazepam, oxazepam, and tybamate—over an inactive placebo.

In the case of meprobamate, for example, Rickels and Snow[22] found that it was definitely more effective in the treatment of the moderately to mildly anxious neurotic patients than placebo (or even phenobarbital). Yet in a further analysis of this study Shader[23] noted that when the psychiatric and medical patients were kept separate the use of meprobamate was not significantly better than placebo at the 5 percent level in the psychiatric patients on physicians' ratings of anxiety, depression, irritability, or headache. Only for insomnia relief was meprobamate superior ($p < 0.02$) to placebo.

Klein and Davis[24] provided definitive evidence that at least the most frequently employed minor tranquilizers do have a therapeutic effect. They presented "box scores" based on the comparative effectiveness of six minor tranquilizers with placebo in 97 double-blind controlled studies. They found that in most studies barbiturates or meprobamate were more effective than placebo (11 out of 17 and 16 out of 25 studies, respectively). Furthermore, out of 13 studies, diazepam was found to be statistically better than placebo in 11, and out of nine studies, oxazepam was found to be significantly superior than an inactive preparation in eight. In all of 22 studies reviewed chlordiazepoxide was significantly better than placebo. The same applies to the 11 studies reviewed on tybamate.

For some time it has been seriously considered that differences among the clinically used minor tranquilizers are slight or absent, at least insofar as overall therapeutic efficacy is concerned. More recently, however, there are indications that there are some differences among the overall therapeutic efficacies of at least some of the minor tranquilizers. For instance, it has been shown in double-blind controlled studies that most minor tranquilizers are more effective (seven studies) than or equal to (18 studies) barbiturates. Out of six studies, diazepam was found to be statistically significantly better than barbiturates in three; out of seven studies, chlordiazepoxide was significantly better in three, and out of 12 studies, meprobamate produced significantly more improvement in one.[24] Furthermore, Rickels[25] asserts that, in most controlled studies which report no statistically significant differences between minor tranquilizers and barbiturates, simple inspection of data gives the following rank order of drug efficacy: (1) minor tranquilizers, (2) phenobarbital sodium or amobarbital sodium, and (3) placebo.

Do Anxiolytic Sedatives Differ in Their Action?

The slight improvement in overall therapeutic efficacy with the new drugs does not justify the rather large number of clinically available minor tranquilizers. Nevertheless, if the new minor tranquilizers would qualitatively differ in their therapeutic action from the older ones, this alone would justify their existence.

It was considered that acute patients—independent of diagnosis and nature of anxiety—responded best to barbiturate treatment whereas chronic patients did not respond to it. Supporting data for this contention were obtained in a study by Rickels et al.,[26] who found that patients with acute symptoms (6 months or less) responded comparatively best to phenobarbital (and also to placebo), but that meprobamate and chlordiazepoxide seemed to be superior to phenobarbital (and also to placebo) in patients with chronic symptoms. Similar findings were reported by Jenner et al.[27,28] and Wheatley.[29]

Rickels in 1967 presented a comprehensive review of the pharmacotherapy of anxiety and tension.[25] He pointed out important relationships between psychopathological symptom profiles and responsiveness to specific pharmacotherapeutic agents. At first, Overall et al.[30] demonstrated that depressed patients could be subdivided into three symptom profiles: anxious-depressed, hostile-depressed, and retarded-depressed; and they observed that a large number of depressed patients, namely, anxious-depressed and hostile-depressed patients, did better with the neuroleptic thioridazine than with the tricyclic antidepressant imipramine, whereas imipramine was most affective in the nonanxious, retarded-depressed patients. More recently Hollister et al.[31] reported similar differential results for perphenazine, a neuroleptic phenothiazine, and amitriptyline, a tricyclic antidepressant.

Whereas Overall et al.[30] found neuroleptics (major tranquilizers) therapeutically effective in anxious-depressed patients, Rickels et al.[32] found minor tranquilizers useful for the same group. In their study, meprobamate produced as much symptomatic improvement in depressed neurotic outpatients as did protriptyline, a tricyclic antidepressant with no antianxiety properties. In fact, during the first 2-week study period, meprobamate caused significantly more symptom reduction than protriptyline. By dividing depressed neurotic patients into high and low anxious groups, in further analysis they found that low anxious-depressed patients improved most and high-anxious depressed patients least with protriptyline, and the latter patients improved most with meprobamate or a combination of meprobamate and protriptyline.

Rickels et al.[33] found another symptom dimension of prognostic value: the dimension of emotional (psychological) versus somatic symptom focus. Applying this dimension in the analysis of data they were able to demonstrate that deprol, a combination of meprobamate and benactyzine, was more effective in somatizing, anxious-depressed patients than imipramine, whereas imipramine was more effective in less anxious, less somatizing depressed patients. In the same frame of reference fluphenazine, in anxious as well as depressed patients, produced significantly poorer results in somatizing medical clinical than in less somatizing, more emotionally focused general practice patients.[21,34] It was also demonstrated that meprobamate alone and chlordiazepoxide alone were about equally effective in both somatic and emotional neurotic symptoms.[33,35,36] Tybamate was most effective in patients with a somatic symptom focus. Diazepam and phenobarbital, on the other hand, seemed to be slightly more effective in patients displaying emotional symptom focus.[25]

Using an entirely different framework, Feldman[37] was able to show differences among the three most frequently employed benzodiazepine preparations. Anxiety reduction was approximately the same with the three compounds, but when hostility was considered, chlordiazepoxide produced a 7 percent improvement, diazepam produced no improvement, and oxazepam was associated with a 50-percent improvement rate. If hypoactivity was considered, chlordiazepoxide, diazepam, and oxazepam produced improvement rates of 0 percent, 36 percent, and 12 percent, respectively, and if hyperactivity was considered, the rates were 46 percent, 0 percent, and 39 percent, respectively. These findings were supported by Shader,[23] who found that the use of chlordiazepoxide and diazepam was associated with increased hostility levels in normal male volunteer subjects whereas the use of oxazepam did not produce such hostility increments. On the basis of these data, Shader[23] suggests that for the inhibited, motor-retarded, but anxious patient, diazepam may be the ideal drug; for the overactive anxious patient, chlordiazepoxide may be preferable; and for the anxious patient with a history of hostile outbursts or temper tantrums, oxazepam may be the drug of choice.

Practical Considerations

Suicide

The rate of suicidal attempts made with any drug prescribed for neurotic or depressed patients increases with the number of years the drug has been on the market; it may be only a question of time when suicidal attempts will be made as frequently with other drugs as they are made now with barbiturates. In the meantime, the fact that barbiturates are among the most toxic of all psychotherapeutic drugs should be fully realized. Some drugs, e.g., chlordiazepoxide (CDZ) or the benzodiazepines in general, seem to be almost suicide proof to the extent that suicidal attempts with as high a dosage as 2250 mg. of CDZ remained unsuccessful. Other minor tranquilizers like the propanediols in general, or meprobamate in particular, can produce fatal poisoning, but are, nevertheless, safer than the barbiturates. Still less toxic are the neuroleptics. Therefore, in consideration of the danger of possible suicide, a physician might sometimes prescribe neuroleptics rather than minor tranquilizers, in spite of the fact that neuroleptics are less effective in reducing anxiety than minor tranquilizers.

Driving

In spite of considerable investigative effort devoted to the question of the interaction of minor tranquilizers with driving skill and performance, the evidence reported in different studies is still conflicting. There is general agreement, however, that the combination of even moderate doses of alcohol with minor tranquilizers produces significant impairment of the judgment and skills necessary to drive a car. Kielholz et al.[38] showed in a carefully designed and conducted study that single therapeutic doses of minor tranquilizers did not significantly impair driving performance unless the drugs were combined with alcohol. However, in the same experiment, alcohol alone impaired driving performance as much as it did in combination with drugs.

Theoretical Considerations

Pharmacotherapy of anxiety may be rendered somewhat less complex if anxiety is viewed in terms of three essential components.

The first component, arousal, is a diffuse and fundamental property of all behavior and it is mainly responsible for the intensity of anxiety. Physiologically it is a function of the reticular ascending system (RAS). The second factor, affect, refers to the specific qualities of feeling, behavior, and somatic response which characterize anxiety. It is now generally accepted that affects are elaborated in the limbic system, which is responsible for the interpretation of all personal experience in subjective terms of feeling. The third component is apperception, i.e., articulate awareness and cognitive evaluation of any affective experience, a function of the neocortex.

All three components—RAS, limbic lobe, and neocortex—are involved in the subjective experience of anxiety, forming a mutual feedback network. Barbiturates inhibit this entire feedback network in a nonselective, global manner.[39] The newer minor tranquilizers have less inhibitory effect on the RAS and on the neocortex. They exert most of their inhibitory action on the limbic system.[40,41] The neuroleptics sometimes, but not always, inhibit the RAS and have even less inhibitory effect on the neocortex than the newer minor tranquilizers. Neuroleptics also effect the limbic system in a way which differs from the minor tranquilizers; the neuroleptics tend to increase the activity of some limbic structures, e.g., the hippocampus. Increased limbic system activity, induced by neuroleptics, is associated with a slowing of the cortical EEG; on the other hand, decreased limbic system activity, induced by minor tranquilizers, is associated with a faster EEG, which is also characterized by a lower energy content.[42,43]

On the biochemical level there is increasing evidence that plasma and urinary catecholamine levels are elevated in anxious patients[44,45] with a subsequent rise in nonesterified fatty acid concentration in the blood and with an increase in the urinary output of hippuric acid.[46] Because of this it is important that most minor tranquilizers decrease catecholamines or antagonize their effects.

An entirely new concept in the treatment of anxiety was presented by the introduction of propranolol,[47] a beta-receptor blocking agent[48] which was shown to be useful in the treatment of neurotic patients with manifest anxiety and cardiac symptoms, e.g., tachycardia.[49,50] Whether the anxiolytic effects[51,52] of propranolol are due to its peripheral action, i.e., interference with physical abnormalities which result in anxiety,[53] or to direct central effects, as has been suggested by Leszkovsky and Tardos,[54] still remains to be seen.

Heuristically most important, however, is that anxiety can be artificially induced by a variety of drugs with well-defined chemical structures and pharmacological actions. Under the influence of these substances the common and the differential characteristics of anxiety can be studied and the treatment of anxiety can be systematically investigated. A number of drugs have been reported to induce anxiety and/or tension, among them autonomic-sympathomimetics (ephedrine, epinephrine, or amphetamines) and various psychotomimetic substances, among which yohimbine, lysergic acid diethylamide, psilocybin, and mescaline are the most important. Parallel with the increase in anxiety and/or tension, under the influence of these drugs, there is also an increase in nonesterfied free fatty acid concentrations in the blood.[55] There are indications that the high free fatty acid levels can be prevented or counteracted by both somnolent insulin or high doses (3000 mg. per day) of nicotinic acid. Nicotinic acid can also prevent stress-induced mobilization of free fatty acids.

Artificially induced anxiety is perhaps one of the best available methods for the intensive study of specific anxiety and also for the systematic exploration of its specific prevention and/or treatment. But artificially, drug-induced anxieties also present themselves today as clinical conditions with increasing frequency. To understand this developing area of psychiatry and to define its scope and treatments are beyond the topic of minor tranquilizers and are among the great new challenges psychiatry and clinical psychopharmacology will have to meet.

REFERENCES

1. Oxford Dictionary. London, Oxford University Press, 1961.
2. Delay, J., and Deniker, P.: 38 cas de psychoses traités par la cure prolongée et continué de 4568 RP. Ann Medicopsychol. (Paris) 110:364, 1952.
3. Lehmann, H. E., and Hanrahan, G. E.: Chlorpromazine: New Inhibiting Agent for Psychomotor Excitement and Manic States. Arch. Neurol. Psychiat. 71:227, 1954.
4. Kline, N. S.: Use of Rauwolfia Serpentina Benth in Neuropsychiatric Conditions. Ann. N.Y. Acad. Sci. 59:107, 1954.
5. Ban, T. A.: Psychopharmacology. Baltimore, The Williams and Wilkins Company, 1969.
6. Lehmann, H. E., and Ban, T. A.: Pharmacotherapy of Tension and Anxiety. Springfield, Ill., Charles C Thomas, Publisher, 1970.

7. WHO: Report of a Scientific Group on Research in Psychopharmacology. Technical Report Series No. 371, Geneva, 1967.
8. Berger, F. M.: Anxiety and the discovery of the Tranquilizers. In: Ayd, F. J., and Blackwell, B. (Eds.), Discoveries in Biological Psychiatry. Philadelphia, J. B. Lippincott Co., 1970.
9. Berger, F. M., and Bradley, W.: The Pharmacological Properties of a β-Dihydroxy-(2-methylphenoxy)-propane (Myanesin). Brit. J. Pharmacol. 1:265, 1946.
10. Gammon, G. D., and Churchill, J. A.: Effects of Myanesin upon the Central Nervous System. Amer. J. Med. Sci. 217:143, 1949.
11. Schlan, L. S., and Unna, K. R.: Some Effects of Myanesin in Psychiatric Patients. J.A.M.A. 140:672, 1949.
12. Splitter, S. R.: A New Psychotropic Drug: Evaluation of Tybamate in the Treatment of Anxiety and Tension States. Psychosomatics 5:292, 1964.
13. Shelton, J., and Hollister, L. E.: Simulated Abuse of Tybamate in Man. J.A.M.A. 199:338, 1967.
14. Lehmann, J. E.: Tranquilizers, Clinical Insufficiencies and Needs. In: Cerletti, A., and Bové, F. J. (Eds.), The Present Status of Psychotropic Drugs. Amsterdam, Excerpta Medica Foundation, 1968.
15. Silver, D., Beaubien, J., Ban, T. A., Saxena, B. M., and Bennett, Jean: Hydroxyzine, Amitriptyline and Their Combination in the Treatment of Psychoneurotic Patients. Curr. Ther. Res. 11:663, 1969.
16. Beaubien, J., Ban, T. A., Lehmann, H. E., and Jarrold, Louise: Doxepin in the Treatment of Psychoneurotic Patients. Curr. Ther. Res. 12(4):192, 1970.
17. Sterlin, C., Ban, T. A., Lehmann, H. E., and Jarrold, Louise: A Comparative Evaluation of Doxepin and Chlordiazepoxide in the Treatment of Psychoneurotic Outpatients. Curr. Ther. Res. 12(4):195, 1970.
18. Lorr, M., McNair, D. M., Weinstein, G. J., Michaux, W. W., and Raskin, A.: Meprobamate and Chlorpromazine in Psychotherapy. Some Effects on Anxiety and Hostility of Outpatients. Arch. Gen. Psychiat. (Chicago) 4:381, 1961.
19. Lorr, M., McNair, D. M., and Weinstein, J.: Early Effects of Chlordiazepoxide (Librium) Used with Psychotherapy. J. Psychiat. Res. 1:257, 1963.
20. Caffey, E. M., Hollister, L., Klett, C. J., and Kaim, S. C.: Veterans Administration (VA) Cooperative Studies in Psychiatry. In: Clark, W. G., and del Giudice, J. (Eds.), Principles of Psychopharmacology. New York, Academic Press, Inc., 1970.
21. Rickels, K., Raab, E., Gordon, P. E., Laquer, K. G., DeSilverio, R. V., and Hesbacher, P.: Differential Effects of Chlordiazepoxide and Fluphenazine in Two Anxious Patient Populations. Psychopharmacologia (Berlin) 12:181, 1968.
22. Rickels, K., and Snow, L.: Meprobamate and Phenobarbital Sodium in Anxious Neurotic Psychiatric and Medical Clinical Outpatients. A Controlled Study. Psychopharmacologia (Berlin) 5:339, 1964.
23. Shader, R. I.: Antianxiety Agents: A Clinical Perspective: In: Dimascio, A., and Shader, R. I. (Eds.), Clinical Handbook of Psychopharmacology. New York, Science House, 1970.
24. Klein, D. F., and Davis, J. M.: Diagnosis and Drug Treatment of Psychiatric Disorders. Baltimore, The Williams and Wilkins Co., 1969.
25. Rickels, K.: Antineurotic Agents: Specific and Non-specific Effects. In: Efron, D. H. (Ed.), Psychopharmacology: A Review of Progress. Washington, Public Health Service Publication No. 1836, 1968.
26. Rickels, K., Clark, T. W., Ewing, J. H., Klingensmith, W. C., Morris, H. M., and Smock, C. D.: Evaluation of Tranquilizing Drugs in Medical Outpatients. Meprobamate, Prochlorperazine, Amobarbital Sodium and Placebo. J.A.M.A. 171:1649, 1959.

27. Jenner, F. A., Kerry, R. J., and Parkin, D.: A Controlled Trial of Methaminodiazepoxide (Chlordiazepoxide, "Librium") in the Treatment of Anxiety in Neurotic Patients. J. Ment. Sci. 107:575, 1961.
28. Jenner, F. A., Kerry, R. J., and Parkin, D.: A Controlled Comparison of Methaminodiazepoxide (Chlordiazepoxide, "Librium") and Amylobarbitone in the Treatment of Anxiety in Neurotic Patients. J. Ment. Sci. 107:583, 1961.
29. Wheatley, D.: Chlordiazepoxide in the Treatment of the Domiciliary Case of Anxiety Neurosis. In: Proceedings of the Fourth World Congress of Psychiatry. Amsterdam, Excerpta Medica Foundation, 1968.
30. Overall, J. E., Hollister, L. E., Meyer, F., Kimbell, I., and Shelton, J.: Imipramine and Thioridazine in Depressed and Schizophrenic Patients. J.A.M.A. 189:605, 1964.
31. Hollister, L. E., Overall, J. E., Shelton, J., Pennington, V., Kimbell, I., and Johnson, M.: Drug Therapy of Depression. Arch. Gen. Psychiat. (Chicago) 17:486, 1967.
32. Rickels, K., Raab, E., DeSilverio, R. V., and Etemad, B.: Drug Treatment in Depression: Antidepressant or Tranquilizer? J.A.M.A. 201:675, 1967.
33. Rickels, K., Ward, C. H., and Schut, L.: Different Populations, Different Drug Responses. Amer. J. Med. Sci. 247:328, 1964.
34. Rickels, K., Snow, L., Uhlenhuth, E. H., Lipman, R. S., Park, L. C., and Fisher, S.: Side Reactions of Meprobamate and Placebo. Dis. Nerv. Syst. 28:39, 1967.
35. Rickels, K., Baumm, C., Raab, E., Taylor, W., and Moore, E.: A Psychopharmacological Evaluation of Chlordiazepoxide, LA-1 and Placebo, Carried out with Anxious Neurotic Medical Clinic Patients. Med. Times 93:238, 1965.
36. Rickels, K., Downing, R. W., and Downing, M. H.: Personality Differences Between Somatically and Psychologically Oriented Neurotic Patients. J. Nerv. Ment. Dis. 142:10, 1966.
37. Feldman, P. E.: Current Views on Antianxiety Agents. Pamphlet from Scientific Exhibit presented at the Annual Meeting of the American Medical Association, Houston, Texas, 1967.
38. Kielholz, P., Goldberg, L., Obersteg, J., Poeldinger, W., Ramsay, A., and Schmid, P.: Circulation routière, tranquillisants et alcohol. Hyg. Ment. 2:39, 1967.
39. Aston, R., and Domino, E. F.: Differential Effects of Phenobarbital, Pentobarbital and Diphenylhydantoin on Motor Cortical and Reticular Thresholds in the Rhesus Monkey. Psychopharmacologia (Berlin) 2:304, 1961.
40. Kletzkin, M., and Berger, F. M.: Effect of Certain Tranquilizers in the Reticular Endothetical System. Proc. Soc. Exp. Biol. Med. 102:88, 1959.
41. Schallek, W., Zabransky, F., and Kuehn, A.: Effects of Benzodiazepines on the Central Nervous System of the Cat. Arch. Int. Pharmacodyn. 149:467, 1964.
42. Itil, T. M.: Electroencephalography and Pharmacopsychiatry. In: Freyhan, F. A., Petrilowitsch, N., and Pichot, P. (Eds.), Clinical Psychopharmacology. Basel, Karger, 1968.
43. Pfeiffer, C. C., Goldstein, L., Murphee, H. B., and Jenney, E. M.: Electroencephalographic Assay of Anti-anxiety Drugs. Arch. Gen. Psychiat. 10:446, 1964.
44. Woolfson, G.: Recent Advances in the Anxiety States. In: Coppen, A., and Walk, A. (Eds.), Recent Developments in Affective Disorders. Ashford, Headley Brothers Ltd., 1968.
45. Levi, L.: Neuro-endocrinology of Anxiety. In: Lader, M. H. (Ed.), Studies of Anxiety. Ashford, Headley Brothers Ltd., 1969.
46. Sourkes, T. L.: Biochemical Changes in the Expression of Emotion. Canad. Psychiat. Ass. J. 7:529, 1962.
47. Turner, P. G., Grossman, K. L., and Smart, J. V.: Effect of Adrenergic Receptor

    Blockade on the Tachycardia of Thyrotoxicosis and Anxiety States. Lancet 2:1316,
    1965.
48. Ahlquist, R. P.: Study of Adrenotropic Receptors. Amer. J. Physiol. 153:586, 1948.
49. Besterman, E. M. M., and Friedlander, D. H.: Clinical Experiences with Propranolol.
    Postgrad. Med. 41:426, 1965.
50. Nordenfeldt, O.: Orthostatic ECG Changes and the Adrenergic Beta Receptor Blocking
    Agent Propranolol (Inderal). Acta Med. Scand. 178:393, 1965.
51. Grossman, G. K. L., and Turner, F.: The Effect of Propranolol in Anxiety. Lancet
    1:788, 1966.
52. Wheatley, D.: Comparative Effects of Propranolol and Chlordiazepoxide in Anxiety.
    Brit. J. Psychiat. 115:1411, 1969.
53. Frohlich, E. D., Dustan, H. P., and Page, I. H.: Hyperdynamic Adrenergic Circulatory
    State. Arch. Int. Med. 117:614, 1966.
54. Leszkovsky, G., and Tardos, L.: Some Effects of Propranolol on the Central Nervous
    System. J. Pharm. Pharmacol. 17:518, 1965.
55. Hollister, L. E.: Drug-Induced Psychoses and Schizophrenic Reactions: A Critical
    Comparison. Ann. N.Y. Acad. Sci. 96:80, 1962.

Optimum Use of Antipsychotic Drugs

by Leo E. Hollister, M.D.

Although the disaster that is schizophrenia has been partially mitigated by drugs, our knowledge of the pathophysiological mechanisms of this disorder is still meager. The impetus provided by the success of drugs in treating this disorder resulted in many inquiries into the biological bases for it. Older notions that schizophrenia is a "functional" disorder based on social-psychological influences have fewer adherents. The present tendency is to regard schizophrenia as a genetically determined disorder whose phenotypic expression may be influenced in part by life experiences. As antischizophrenic drugs were discovered fortuitously, our continuing lack of knowledge of the pathogenesis of the disorder has limited development of more effective drugs. We have new chemicals, but old drugs.

Chemical Structures

Seven chemical classes of drugs have the two unique pharmacological properties of neuroleptic or antipsychotic drugs: the ability to ameliorate schizophrenia and to evoke extrapyramidal syndromes. The structures of most antipsychotic drugs can be viewed as tertiary, or rarely secondary, amines derived from methylamine (–C–C–N–C). Phenothiazine antipsychotics have the following common S-shaped configuration, regardless of the subfamily to which they belong (R–N–C–C–C–N–C). Thioxanthenes are similar, as are the butyrophenones (R–C–C–C–C–N–C).[1] Presumably this S shape is crucial to the fit of the molecule with its receptor, although an adequate model of the receptor for antipsychotic drugs has not yet been proposed. For practical purposes we are concerned with only three chemical classes: phenothiazines, thioxanthenes, and butyrophenones, the first two having strong chemical resemblances to each other. The members of these classes are listed in Table 1, which shows those drugs presently available in the United States.

Pharmacological Properties

The aliphatic phenothiazines are highly sedative, with strong adrenergic blocking actions. Thus they are most useful in patients for whom some sedative

81

TABLE 1

Antipsychotic Drugs Available in the United States

	Estimated Equivalent Dose (mg.)
Phenothiazines	
Aliphatic	
Chlorpromazine (Thorazine)	100
Triflupromazine (Vesprin)	25
Piperidine	
Thioridazine (Mellaril)	100
Piperacetazine (Quide)	10
Piperazine	
Acetophenazine (Tindal)	20
Butaperazine (Repoise)	10
Carphenazine (Proketazine)	25
Fluphenazine (Prolixin)	2
Perphenazine (Trilafon)	10
Prochlorperazine (Compazine)	15
Thiopropazate (Dartal)	10
Trifluoperazine (Stelazine)	5
Thioxanthenes	
Chlorprothixene (Taractan)	100
Thiothixene (Navane)	4
Butyrophenone	
Haloperidol (Haldol)	2

effect is desirable. The piperidine derivative thioridazine is similar to the aliphatic derivatives in its sedative and adrenergic blocking action. Like the aliphatics, thioridazine would be considered a "high-dose" phenothiazine. Unlike the other phenothiazines, thioridazine has little tendency to produce extrapyramidal effects and is devoid of antiemetic action. Its peripheral adrenergic blocking action is the greatest of all these drugs.

The piperazine group of phenothiazines may be considered as low-dose drugs owing to their greater potency. Although they are often claimed to have an "activating" action, this may be spurious. They are less overtly sedative in the usual therapeutic doses than the others. They also tend to increase the motor activity of patients, but this is usually a purposeless, driven, and highly uncomfortable side effect termed akathisia.

The thioxanthenes also share many of the same properties as the phenothiazines. One derivative, chlorprothixene, may be considered a high-dose drug, whereas the other, thiothixene, is a low-dose drug. Haloperidol, the butyrophenone derivative, is also quite potent, with strong tendencies to evoke extrapyramidal syndromes and akathisia.

Because the antipsychotic effects of "low-dose" drugs are greater in proportion to their sedative or peripheral autonomic effects, the French have termed them *"neuroleptique incisif,"* or what we may call a "specific antipsychotic."

Clinical Efficacy of Antipsychotics

Well-controlled studies from many sources indicate that most of these drugs effectively control symptoms of schizophrenia, allowing the rehabilitation of many patients who appeared doomed to a lifetime of hospitalization. The relationship of drug therapy to the practice of psychiatry as well as the balance between therapeutic and side effects has been reviewed elsewhere.[2]

With the exception of mepazine and promazine, both of which are too weak in antipsychotic action to justify their hazards, the phenothiazine derivatives have been repeatedly found to be equally efficacious when the responses of groups of patients have been compared.[3-6] The efficacy of these drugs has been proven in every kind of schizophrenic patient, from those suffering their initial schizophrenic symptoms to those who had been exiled to hospitals for years. It is regrettable, in retrospect, that so much time, talent, and money were expended to prove what should have been obvious to any unbiased clinician who treated several schizophrenics with these drugs: something new and different and exciting was happening. Still, the effort has at least refined the methodology for studying the effects of treatments for schizophrenia to such an extent that it is now beginning to be possible to evaluate others in the same precise way that drugs have been studied.

The Question of Specific Indications

Despite their overall efficacy, individual patients respond differently to these drugs, doing poorly on some and better on others. The more sedative phenothiazines, such as chlorpromazine and thioridazine, were thought initially to be preferable for patients with agitation; less sedative drugs, such as trifluoperazine and perphenazine, were considered best for patients with symptoms of withdrawal and retardation. This rough dichotomy between "active" and "inactive" patients still forms the primary basis for choice of drugs.

A few systematic approaches to the problem have been attempted with uncertain results. Classification of schizophrenic patients into empirically derived subtypes on the basis of initial signs and symptoms, derivation of regression equations to distinguish clusters of symptoms responding to different drugs, and using clinically determined distinctions have all had the usual history of first revealing possible differences between drugs which later failed to be replicated.[7,8]

The latest review of the entire subject of predicting responses to antipsychotic drugs by one of the participants of these studies concluded that the present evidence for a differential action of antipsychotic drugs was highly inconclusive.[9] This conclusion seems eminently reasonable, especially when one considers that the various schizophrenic groupings were based on retrospective analysis of group data; the proper choice of drug in advance for individual patients would be a vastly greater problem.

Choice of Antipsychotic Drug in the Clinic

The wide array of antipsychotic drugs available for clinicians in the United States has been shown in Table 1, which lists 15. A choice must be made from this bewildering array of drugs of one to be given an empirical trial in a given patient. The usual dictum for dealing with a multiplicity of similar drugs has been to learn to use a few drugs well rather than all poorly. The differences between the proper and improper use of a drug will probably exceed any actual difference between drugs. One of the most rational ways to narrow the choice of antipsychotics would be to master one of each of the three types of phenothiazines, one of the two thioxanthenes, and a butyrophenone.

Making a choice of five drugs is not all that difficult. Chlorpromazine is the logical choice among aliphatic phenothiazines, simply because of its great familiarity and popularity. Thioridazine is unique in the piperidine group of phenothiazines, as piperacetazine is only technically a piperidine, resembling the piperazines in structural geometry and pharmacological actions. Any of the piperazine group could be selected, based mainly on one's familiarity with the drug. Thiothixene is probably the preferred thioxanthene, owing primarily to its greater potency. Haloperidol is the only available butyrophenone. With five drugs chosen on this basis, one should be able to exploit the full range of pharmacological differences between the various antipsychotics.

Special Considerations in Choosing for Specific Patients

The patient's past performance is a quite reliable guide. If he has done well previously on some drug, and especially if he has done less well on others, one could be foolhardy to change drugs or to reinstitute lapsed treatment with a different drug. To the objective response of the patient must also be added his subjective response. Unless a patient tolerates a drug well, he is not likely to maintain treatment faithfully. A patient who is made unbearably restless by a drug may much prefer no drug. On the other hand, some patients may prefer restlessness rather than impairment of their sexual capacity. The importance of various side effects to the patient should be a guide in choosing his specific treatment.

Although high-dose drugs, such as chlorpromazine and thioridazine, are more sedative than low-dose drugs, sedation is not the most wanted effect. Antipsychotic drugs should be used to treat symptoms of schizophrenia. It may be better to rely on conventional sedatives, hypnotics, or antianxiety drugs to manage excited states, anxiety, or sleeplessness. Sedation alone should not dictate the choice of antipsychotic drug, although if the combination of effects is appropriate, so much the better.

Many clinicians seem to prefer to choose two or more drugs in combination rather than using only one. In fact, in reviewing an order for a patient, one frequently finds the following conglomeration: two phenothiazines (one high-dose and one low-dose); a tricyclic antidepressant (the patient is withdrawn); an antiparkinson drug (even if the patient has never shown any signs; this drug is completely superfluous in the presence of the anticholinergic tricyclic antidepressant); something for sleep; and something during the day to keep the patient awake. Such a choice of drugs is no choice at all and has many irrational aspects. Small wonder that some patients seem to improve after drugs are withdrawn! A fair number of systematic studies of drug combinations have now been completed, with no convincing evidence that any combination is superior for treating schizophrenics than a properly chosen single drug.[10]

Some patients may tolerate antipsychotic drugs so poorly that no drug treatment should be given. As these patients tend to be less psychotic than most schizophrenics, with retention of insight and marked somatization, it may be that they represent a "schizophreniform" group rather than true schizophrenia. One should bear in mind that to take antipsychotic drugs, one must be crazy, either literally or figuratively. The ability to tolerate these drugs seems to be directly correlated with the severity of the psychosis.

Specific Problems in the Use of Antipsychotics

Few drugs have such great therapeutic margins and such a wide range of therapeutic doses as these. Differences in daily doses of 20- to 30-fold have been recorded. Requirements of most patients fall within a narrower range, usually from 200 to 800 mg. daily based on chlorpromazine doses. Occasional patients may do well with higher doses. Although no patient should be considered a drug failure without an intensive course of therapy, routine use of massive doses may represent overtreatment for many. As measurement of plasma concentrations of these drugs is far from being a suitable laboratory control for dose, one must rely on clinical signs. The unique pharmacological effects of antipsychotic drugs are amelioration of schizophrenia and production of extrapyramidal syndromes, probably both mediated through dopaminergic system blockade. If neither of these signs has become clinically evident, I would be reluctant to believe that the patient had received an adequate dose of drug at the receptor sites in brain that we want to reach.

Until comparatively recently, not much attention was given to the bio-pharmaceutical preparation of these drugs. A recent study indicates that the biological availability of drug may be far greater in some dosage forms than in others.[11] Chlorpromazine was most reliably given by intramuscular injection, where plasma levels were uniformly and promptly attained; the intramuscular dose was about four times as potent as the same dose given orally. Oral preparations were by no means totally reliable, liquid concentrates being somewhat better than coated tablets. Delayed-action preparations were the least reliable, and of dubious need in the case of drugs which are highly cumulative. Failure of a patient to respond adequately may be less the fault of the drug than of its dosage form; a brief trial of parenteral administration followed by maintenance with liquid concentrate might be tried in such patients prior to switching to another drug.

Duration of treatment is an unsettled question. Acute responses of patients newly treated with drugs are variable, ranging from days to weeks. Most clinicians would feel that failure of acute or newly admitted schizophrenics to improve after 6 to 8 weeks of adequate treatment with a drug would be reason to try another. Newly treated chronic patients might require 12 to 24 weeks of treatment before a change of medication would be warranted. Improvement tends to be more rapid earlier than later on, when therapeutic gains creep.

Assuming that complete or partial remission is attained, how long should treatment be continued? As far as one can tell, it should probably be indefinitely for most patients. The consequence of replacing drug with placebo in stabilized hospitalized patients revealed a linear rate of clinical relapse over a 4-month period, affecting 45 percent of these patients.[12] Of considerable interest was the fact that a sharp reduction in maintenance doses to three-sevenths of those usually given resulted in only a 15 percent relapse rate over the same period. Apparently, many patients receive higher-than-necessary maintenance doses of drug. Still, it might be argued that 55 percent of patients remain in clinical remission after being off drug for a substantial period and that "drug holidays" might be in order. The difficulty is that, despite the most earnest attempts, patients who maintained improvement could not be distinguished from those who relapsed. Consequently, the most practical approach would be to consider definite uninterrupted treatment for most patients. The consequences of doing otherwise are quite evident; lapses in maintenance therapy with antipsychotic drugs are presently the most frequent cause of readmission to a mental hospital following discharge. On the other side of the coin, the value of phenothiazines in preventing psychiatric hospitalization seems to be well established.[13]

General Principles

1. Antipsychotic drugs should be used primarily for treating symptoms of schizophrenia and not for trivial purposes (such as sleep disturbance or excitement) better treated with other drugs.

2. A rational choice can be made from the many available drugs based on chemical and pharmacological differences between groups.

3. Choice of drug for individual patients is still more of an art than a science. Generally "high-dose" drugs are used when behavioral or mood disturbances predominate and "low-dose," specific antipsychotics are employed where thinking disorder predominates.

4. Doses are determined by clinical signs of the patient's response, based on the amelioration of schizophrenia or appearance of extrapyramidal effects.

5. Dosage should best be on an indefinite basis, although brief interruptions are tolerable.

6. One must watch the dosage form of drug to assure that the putative doses actually reach the patient.

REFERENCES

1. Janssen, P. A. J.: Chemical and pharmacological classification of neuroleptics. In: Bobon, D. P., Janssen, P. A. J., and Bobon, J. (Eds.), Modern Problems of Pharmacopsychiatry. Vol. 5. The Neuroleptics. Basel, S. Karger, 1970, pp. 33-44.
2. Kinross-Wright, J.: The Current Status of Phenothiazines. J.A.M.A. 200:461-464, 1967.
3. Casey, J. F., Bennett, I. F., Lindley, C. J., Hollister, L. E., Gordon, M. H., and Springer, N. N.: Drug Therapy in Schizophrenia: A Controlled Study of the Relative Effectiveness of Chlorpromazine, Promazine, Phenobarbital, and Placebo. Arch. Gen. Psychiat. 2:210-220, 1960.
4. Casey, J. F., Lasky, J. J., Klett, C. J., and Hollister, L. E.: Treatment of Schizophrenic Reactions with Phenothiazine Derivatives: A Comparative Study of Chlorpromazine, Triflupromazine, Mepazine, Prochlorperazine, Perphenazine, and Phenobarbital. Amer. J. Psychiat. 117:97-105, 1960.
5. Lasky, J. J., Klett, C. J., Caffey, E. M., Jr., Bennett, J. L., Rosenblum, M. P., and Hollister, L. E.: Drug Treatment of Schizophrenic Patients: A Comparative Evaluation of Chlorpromazine, Chlorprothixene, Fluphenazine, Reserpine, Thioridazine, and Triflupromazine. Dis. Nerv. Syst. 23:698-706, 1962.
6. National Inst. of Mental Health, Psychopharmacol. Service Cen. Collaborative Study Gp.: Phenothiazine Treatment in Acute Schizophrenia. Arch. Gen. Psychiat. 10:246-261, 1964.
7. Hollister, L. E., Overall, J. E., Bennett, J. L., Kimbell, I., Jr., and Shelton, J.: Specific Therapeutic Actions of Acetophenazine, Perphenazine and Benzquinamide in Newly Admitted Schizophrenic Patients. Clin. Pharmacol. Ther. 8:249-255, 1967.
8. Galbrecht, C. R., and Klett, C. J.: Predicting Response to Phenothiazines: The Right Drug for the Right Patient. J. Nerv. Ment. Dis. 147:173-183, 1968.
9. Goldberg, S. C.: Prediction of Response to Anti-psychotic Drugs. In: D. Efron (Ed.), Psychopharmacology. A Review of Progress, 1957-1967. Washington, D.C., U.S. Govt. Printing Office, Public Health Service Publication No. 1836, 1968, pp. 1101-1118.
10. Casey, J. F., Hollister, L. E., Lasky, J. J., Klett, C. J., and Caffey, E. M.: Combined Drug Therapy of Chronic Schizophrenics: A Controlled Evaluation of Placebo, Dextroamphetamine, Imipramine, Isocarboxazid, and Trifluoperazine Added to Maintenance Doses of Chlorpromazine. Amer. J. Psychiat. 117:997-1003, 1961.

11. Hollister, L. E., Curry, S. H., Derr, J. E., and Kanter, S. L.: Studies of Delayed-Action Medication. V. Plasma Levels and Urinary Excretion of Four Different Forms of Chlorpromazine. Clin. Pharmacol. Ther. 11:49-59, 1970.
12. Caffey, E. M., Jr., Diamond, L. S., Frank, T. V., Grasberger, J. C., Herman, L., Klett, C. J., and Rothstein, C.: Discontinuation or Reduction of Chemotherapy in Chronic Schizophrenics. J. Chron. Dis. 17:347-358, 1964.
13. Engelhardt, D. M., Rosen, B., Freedman, N., and Margolis, R.: Phenothiazines in Prevention of Psychiatric Hospitalization. IV. Delay or Prevention of Hospitalization—A Re-evaluation. Arch. Gen. Psychiat. 16:98-101, 1967.

Polypharmacy in Psychiatry: Empiricism, Efficacy, and Rationale*

*by Sidney Merlis, M.D., Virginia Beyel, R.N., Diane Fiorentino, B.A.,
John Fracchia, M.A., and Charles Sheppard, M.A.*

Polypharmacy in psychiatric treatment consists of any combination of major tranquilizing, minor tranquilizing or antidepressant-stimulant medication or both, used in treatment of mental illness. Our purpose here is to review and summarize the results of our completed studies and indicate future directions.

Incidence of Polypharmacy

Initial studies of incidence demonstrated that the practice of polypharmacy was not novel. Three of ten hospitalized chronic psychotic patients who were studied received polypharmacy. Half of the polypharmacy prescriptions were for combinations using major tranquilizers. Twenty-nine per cent of the drug combinations consisted of an antidepressant and another psychoactive agent. Minor tranquilizers were used in combination 12 per cent of the time.[8]

Incidence data for geriatric patients indicated a decrease in the combination of major tranquilizer medication to 39 per cent, whereas antidepressant and minor tranquilizer medication in combination increased to 33 and 17 per cent, respectively. In addition to ascertaining incidence data and showing that the types of drugs used in combination change as a function of age, certain other demographic and treatment variables were considered.[1,9]

Female patients received polypharmacy treatment about twice as often as male patients. Female patients were older. The onset of their symptoms occurred earlier in life, and they remained nonhospitalized for a longer duration than male patients who received polypharmacy. When a drug was prescribed in combination for both sexes, females received the medication in significantly higher dosages. The specific drugs used in combination within the three categories of major and minor tranquilizers and antidepressant differed for males and females. For example, chlorpromazine, thioridazine, trifluoperazine, and amitriptyline were prescribed proportionally greater for males. Females were

*This work was supported in part by Public Health Service Grant MH-05096 from the National Institute of Mental Health.

89

treated with chlorprothixine, perphenazine, and imipramine in significantly greater numbers. These data gave us some indication as to what was being prescribed to whom and in what dosage, but did not provide any indication of effectiveness.

Efficacy of Polypharmacy

Questions of the relative effectiveness of polypharmacy were approached from two points of view. A total of 1,350 patients received polypharmacy treatment. A stratified random sample of 500 patients (375 females and 125 males) were selected for evaluation and further study. Selection of patients for further study was conducted on the basis of the proportion of patients treated with polypharmacy by a given psychiatrist. This approach allowed for an unbiased representation of the tendency of each ward psychiatrist to prescribe polypharmacy. The proportion of patients prescribed polypharmacy was represented in the sample drawn from his service. A team of raters, without knowledge of the patient treatment regimen, interviewed and recorded manifest symptomatology on the Brief Psychiatric Rating Scale (BPRS).[4,11] Intraclass correlations measuring the degree of agreement among the six raters on the BPRS items ranged from a low of 0.70 to a high of 0.82, indicating concordance among the different raters, and allowed for pooling of these data for statistical analysis.

In broad terms, patients receiving polypharmacy could be treated with combinations containing two tranquilizers and combinations of a tranquilizer and an antidepressant. For comparative purposes, residual pathology measures were evaluated between male and female patients who received polypharmacy for a 30-day period and who were considered stabilized by their ward psychiatrist.* In addition to the above data, the literature offered sets of data for acute[5] and chronic psychotic patients treated with various marketed single drug forms.[12] Two final groups of patients were added. Male and female chronically ill psychotic patients, treated on the research wards at Central Islip State Hospital, with single drug forms which were deemed as inactive-nontherapeutic, comprise the final comparison group. In all cases cited above, therefore, the patients treated were administered their specific regimen to maximum

*The authors would like to thank the following people from Central Islip State Hospital, Central Islip, N.Y., for their assistance with this study: Drs. Francis J. O'Neill, director, Peter Agola, Fred Allison, Paul Conboy, Richard D'Isernia, Gerardo Espejo, Roman Kernitsky, Andrew May, Mary Mullan, Vivian Roth, John St. Andre, the paramedical staff who made the patients and their treatment records available, and Mrs. Elizabeth Ricca, Kathleen Reinhardt, Elizabeth Ruest, and Annabelle Stipes, members of the Demographic and Special Studies Unit, for their assistance in the various stages of data collection, processing, and statistical analyses.

therapeutic dosage. Mean residual total pathology scores for these groups are seen in Table 1.

Review of the data for patients treated with different types of drug combinations suggests that these differences may be related more to sex of the patient than to treatment differences. Analysis of variance demonstrated no significant differences between females treated with either form of combination treatment. Similarly, where comparison were made between male patients treated with tranquilizer combinations and combinations including an anti-depressant plus a tranquilizer, analysis of variance demonstrated no differences. But when comparisons are made between males and females treated with either

TABLE 1

Mean Residual Total Pathology Scores for Patients
Treated with Polypharmacy and Single-Drug Treatment Forms

Polypharmacy-Treated Patients	Mean Females	Mean Males
Tranquilizer Combinations	45 (N = 167)	39 (N = 71)
Antidepressant-Tranquilizer	45 (N = 218)	40 (N = 44)
Acute Patients		
Acetophenazine[a]		38 (N = 49)
Perphenazine[a]		37 (N = 49)
Chronic Patients		
Nonefficacious Single Drugs[b]	34 (N = 126)	39 (N = 37)
Placebo[c]		34 (N = 28)
Thiothixene[c]		32 (N = 35)
Thioridazine[c]		30 (N = 30)

[a]Data from Ref. 5.
[b]Data recorded at Central Islip State Hospital.
[c]Data from Ref. 12.

combination form, differences in residual pathology scores are significant. The first inference to be drawn from these data suggests a stronger relationship between type of polypharmacy and the patient's sex rather than between type of polypharmacy and remaining symptoms.

It is interesting to note that the remaining residual pathology scores in Table 1, for patients treated with single drug forms, are all lower than polypharmacy-treated patients. This includes samples of acute male psychotic patients treated with acetophenazine or perphenazine, or both. Samples of male chronic psychotic patients treated with single drugs deemed nonefficacious equaled mean residual pathology scores for male patients treated with polypharmacy. Patients treated with placebo, thiothixene, or thioridazine showed lower residual pathology scores than either group of male polypharmacy-treated patients. The one group of female chronic psychotic patients treated with single drugs deemed nonefficacious showed significantly lower residual pathology scores than either group of polypharmacy-treated female patients. These data, while inferential, raised serious questions regarding the efficacy of polypharmacy. Scientific investigation proceeds most effectively by "strong inference," which is pitting alternative hypotheses against one another and putting them to empirical tests. More data collected under controlled conditions was necessary to validate the efficacy of polypharmacy.

The strategy was framed in the following manner: Discounting for the moment the type of polypharmacy the patient received, and using each patient as his own control, one third of all patients were abruptly taken off all active psychiatric medication. Placebos were substituted in a form similar to their usual combination therapy. For a second third of the total group of patients receiving polypharmacy, the ward psychiatrist was instructed to delete what he considered to be the least important medication in the combination. Placebo was substituted in a form similar to the medication discontinued. The remaining third of the patients continued on their usual polypharmacy regimen. All patients remained on the new treatment regimen for a 30-day period and were then rerated. Test-retest reliability coefficients were computed for the six raters by having them rate the same 30 chronic schizophrenic patients who were considered stabilized on a nonpolypharmacy regimen. Pearson product moment coefficients were computed for all BPRS items for each rater between the initial and the second rating completed at the end of 30 days. Coefficients of correlation were converted to Fisher Z scores and summed to establish mean data for the six raters over the BPRS items. These mean reliability coefficients ranged from 0.86 to 0.95, suggesting a high degree of stability within raters over the time period measured. At this point, the rating data showed adequate concordance and stability of the raters, and we could proceed to data analysis and hypothesis testing.

Because of the sex differences in symptom profiles, data for males and females were analyzed separately. Analysis of covariance for multiple covariates was applied to measure the significance of differences in behavioral rating scores. Included as control variables were age, duration of hospital stay, degree of mental illness, total pathology, and first assessment BPRS cluster scores.[6] On the bases of the data seen in Table 1, the following hypotheses were framed: (1) Patients continued on two medications and those shifted to a one-medication and one-placebo regimen will maintain their clinical status. (2) Patients shifted to two placebos will become worse.

The results of the multiple analysis of covariance can be seen in Table 2. Reviewing the data for females first, we found that our hypotheses were supported. Significant differences among the three groups were demonstrated in total pathology, depression, thinking disturbance, and withdrawal retardation. Both patients retained on their combination therapy and those shifted from two medications to one placebo and one medication maintained their clinical status, suggesting no benefit of two active medications over one active medication and one placebo. Patients changed to two placebo showed significant increase in pathology, exceeding their first ratings and also exceeding the symptom levels manifested by the two drug-treated groups. Medication seems to be effective, but two medications are no more effective than one medication for the female patients studied.

Data for male patients indicate that men who were retained on their original individualized combination were more symptomatic than either patients changed to one medication and one placebo or patients changed to a two-placebo regimen. Significant improvement in these latter groups was reflected in lower interpersonal disturbance, depression, withdrawal retardation, and total pathology scores. Insofar as male patients were concerned, polypharmacy appeared to be the least effective form of treatment,[3] but existing conditions, seemingly, lead to polypharmacy.

Rationale for Polypharmacy

One concept underlying the use of psychopolypharmacy is that the more proven a treatment, the better—therefore the tendency to combine two proven medications. Allied with this notion is the support gained from successful treatment utilizing polypharmacy in other areas of medicine. Efficacy of combined drug therapy has been demonstrated in the treatment of tuberculosis and fluid retention states, in psychosomatic disease, in hypertension, and in epilepsy.[2] This success in other areas of medical treatment, when coupled with the present status of drug therapy in psychiatry today, provides a point of departure for adoption of polypharmacy treatment in psychiatry.

Psychopharmacology has reached an impasse in its attempt to develop more effective treatments for mental illness. The psycholeptic properties of current

TABLE 2

Mean Pre- and Covariance Adjusted Post-behavioral Rating Scores for Patients Treated
with Combinations of Placebo and Active Medications

Treatment Regimen	Females				Males			
	Pre	Adjusted Post	F	P	Pre	Adjusted Post	F	P
Two Medication								
Manifest Pathology	44.2	44.1	8.44	0.001	38.3	41.5	3.45	0.01
Thinking Disturbance	13.4	14.6	2.95	0.10	12.4	13.4	2.07	NS
Interpersonal Disturbance	10.9	11.9	.51	NS	10.3	11.3	4.17	0.001
Withdrawal Retardation	13.0	12.7	4.84	0.01	10.4	12.2	2.59	0.05
Depression	13.3	12.3	6.68	0.001	11.7	11.8	2.34	0.05
Placebo-Medication								
Manifest Pathology	44.7	44.5	—	—	40.8	36.8		
Thinking Disturbance	13.9	14.3	—	—	12.2	12.5		
Interpersonal Disturbance	11.4	11.6	—	—	10.2	9.6		
Withdrawal Retardation	13.4	13.1	—	—	12.7	10.2		
Depression	13.2	11.9	—	—	11.1	10.1		
Two Placebo								
Manifest Pathology	42.1	49.3	—	—	38.6	36.3		
Thinking Disturbance	12.8	15.4	—	—	12.7	11.4		
Interpersonal Disturbance	10.7	11.7	—	—	9.8	9.6		
Withdrawal Retardation	13.7	14.4	—	—	11.5	10.5		
Depression	11.4	14.4	—	—	10.4	9.8		

drugs may be characterized as a sophisticated quieting and blunting effect. Available drugs are active in reducing secondary manifestations of mental illness while leaving the core symptoms untouched.[10] Realizing this condition, clinicians may combine drugs with the expectation that the effect of the combination will exceed the potential effects of either drug used singly. Our data suggest this is not the case. In addition to this generally accepted therapeutic effect, antipsychotic drugs produce extrapyramidal symptoms.

With the exception of thioridazine, which elicits fewer extrapyramidal symptoms over a dosage range comparable to that for chlorpromazine, the phenothiazines developed after chlorpromazine are active at lower dosages and produce different side-effect profiles, but avoid the sedative effects of chlorpromazine. Subsequently developed thioxanthenes and butyrophenone derivatives share the same effects of the phenothiazines they mimic. With the availability of a number of antidepressants, minor tranquilizers, and major tranquilizer medications, it could be expected that psychiatric treatment would combine medications on a chance basis.

The addition of medication to the treatment regimen to relieve extrapyramidal and other untoward effects of major tranquilizer therapy soon shifted to the prophylactic use of antiparkinson medication.[7] This in itself reinforces the practice of polypharmacy. Possibly in the face of unremitting symptoms and to avoid undue side effects, the clinician next began to employ two psychoactive drugs in lower dosages to reach a therapeutic response. The practice of combining amitriptyline, desipramine or imipramine, for example, with a major tranquilizer may offer a substitute for the anticholinergic effects of antiparkinson medication. This desire to avoid side effects may serve as some justification for the earlier use of drug combinations. But the more rational approach, it seems, is a careful selection from among the existing drugs, gradually raising dosage of this one drug to its maximum potential as reflected in terms of a therapeutic response or in terms of side-effect incidence.

The practice of combining psychoactive drugs is certainly consistent with the serendipitous discovery of the antipsychotic effects of the first major psychoactive agent, chlorpromazine. However, there are basic realities to treatment choices among the available drugs. Combining these drugs does not seem to be a reasoned choice of treatment.

Finally, the efforts of the pharmaceutical houses should not be overlooked or minimized in the development of polypharmacy in psychiatry. Many continue to capitalize on the present situation. Because we have no fundamental understanding of the pathophysiology of the psychotic process, and because we generally consider schizophrenia a wastebasket diagnosis—comprising a number of syndromes of infinite variety—we attempt to deal with symptoms individually rather than with the disease as a whole through polypharmacy. The influences brought to bear on the clinician in a manner heretofore unexperienced makes the proper use of single drug entities and the careful evaluation of combined drug therapies difficult to accomplish. The availability of numerous psychoactive drugs purported to have special action, the development of prepackaged drug combinations touted as more effective and convenient, the large numbers of patients to be treated, and the aggressive marketing of a seemingly endless variety of psychoactive agents promising efficacy lead the clinician into therapeutic judgments that are not always in the patient's best interest. These may represent some of the factors that contributed to the occurrence of the polypharmacy phenomena. However, the lack of a clear-cut rationale for polypharmacy, coupled with the data presented, raises serious questions regarding the efficacy and continued use of polypharmacy as a treatment choice.

Summary

The present data support the contention that, in terms of incidence, polypharmacy is more than a novel treatment practice. Factors of age, sex, and length of hospitalization are shown to influence the incidence and types of drugs used in combination. The growth of polypharmacy in psychiatry signals a failure of currently available psychoactive agents rather than a new successful development in the treatment of mental disease. Comparative data from several patient groups treated with single drug forms, to include placebo, show single drugs to be the choice of treatment over polypharmacy during a comparable treatment period. Further evaluation of polypharmacy under controlled conditions demonstrate there is no increase in effectiveness over single-drug treatment. Various factors explored have influenced the development of polypharmacy in psychiatry. However, there is no basis in fact for the existence of polypharmacy as a treatment method, nor empirical support for continued use as an efficacious treatment modality. Yet it continues in psychiatry as an aberrant form of drug therapy.

REFERENCES

1. Fracchia, J., Sheppard, C., and Merlis, S.: Polypharmacy in Psychiatric Treatment: Patterns in an Older Patient Group. J. Amer. Geriat. Soc., 1970.
2. Jick, H., and Chalmers, T. C.: Drug Combinations—Uses, Dangers and Fallacies. Clin. Pharmacol. Ther. 6:673-676, 1964.
3. Merlis, S., Sheppard C., Collins, L., and Fiorentino, D.: Polypharmacy in Psychiatry: Patterns of Differential Treatment. Amer. J. Psychiat. 11:1647-1651, 1962.
4. Overall, J., and Gorham, D.: The Brief Psychiatric Rating Scale. Psychol. Rep. 10:799-812, 1962.
5. Overall, J., Hollister, L., Honigfeld, G., Kimbell, I., Jr., Meyer, F., Bennett, J., and Caffey, E., Jr.: Comparison of Acetophenazine with Perphenazine in Schizophrenics: Demonstration of Differential Effects Based on Computer-Derived Diagnostic Models. Clin. Pharmacol. Ther. 4:200-208, 1963.

6. Overall, J., Hollister, L., and Pichot, P.: Major Psychiatric Disorder. Arch. Gen. Psy-hiat. 16:146-151, 1967.
7. Sheppard, C., and Merlis, S.: Drug-Induced Extrapyramidal Symptoms: Their Incidence and Treatment. Amer. J. Psychiat. 7:886-889, 1967.
8. Sheppard, C., Collins, L., Fiorentino, D., Fracchia, J., and Merlis, S.: Polypharmacy in Psychiatric Treatment: I. Incidence at a State Hospital. Curr. Ther. Res. 11:765-774, 1969.
9. Sheppard, C., Fracchia, J., Collins, L., and Merlis, S.: Influences of Polypharmacy on Hallucinatory Behavior in a Sample of Female Chronic Schizophrenic Patients. In: Keup, W. (Ed.), Origin and Mechanisms of Hallucinations. New York, Plenum Publishing Corporation, 1970, pp. 465-470.
10. Sheppard, C., and Merlis, S.: Pragmatic Considerations of Current Models in the Predictors of Psychiatric Drug Effects. Dis. Nerv. Syst. 30:11-14, 1969.
11. Turner, W.: Glossaries for Use with Overall and Gorham Brief Psychiatric Rating Scale. New York, Central Islip State Hospital Press, 1963.
12. Wolpert, A., Sheppard, C., and Merlis, S.: Thiothixene, Thioridazine and Placebo in Male Chronic Schizophrenic Patients. Clin. Pharmacol. Ther. 9:456-464, 1968.

Recent Developments in the Therapy of Addictions

by Paul H. Blachly, M.D.

Drug addiction, unlike most conditions in medicine, is characterized by three primary features: (1) the victim actively engages in his own victimization (he brings it on himself); (2) negativism, or the victim knows the usual consequences of the behavior but does it anyway; (3) a short-term reward and a long-term punishment which is probable but not certain: not every smoker gets lung cancer nor every alcoholic cirrhosis. Addiction, then, is more like gambling, crime, promiscuity, or other risk-taking behaviors than it is like pneumonia, diabetes, or cancer. The distinction is crucial in treatment, for physicians are likely to provide sympathy for the latter conditions and unhelpful moralism or rejection for the former. (The relatively rare patients with iatrogenic addiction constantly point this out to physicians as if it really makes a difference.) Treatment of addiction involves not only the identified patient, but his close contacts and the larger society. Within the identified patient it involves treatment of: (1) drug hunger and drug-seeking behavior such as heroin addiction or alcoholism, (2) the underlying tendency to solve interpersonal problems with drugs (pharma-cothymia), and (3) the complications of drug abuse such as septicemia, psychosis, or cirrhosis.

Although in past times it was customary to think of persons as having a single addiction such as to opium or barbiturates, present experience indicates that patients with such single-minded devotion are exceptional, and that instead we find addicts to be omnivorous, often within the same day taking opiates, barbiturates, alcohol, stimulants, marihuana, and tobacco. Stopping or con-trolling one drug may have little influence on the others, or even stimulate the use of the others.

A further complication is that the doctor's allegiance is more likely to be split between patient, family, and society rather than devoted to the patient alone. Many physicians who treat addicts are government employees, and addicts are coerced into treatment. The expectations of the physician may have little resemblance to the hopes and expectations of the "patient." Unless the physician has a clear understanding of these rather general philosophical dilemmas, he may experience enough unhappiness in treatment of addicts to leave the field for more pleasant pursuits.

One must, then, clearly define at the outset two major factors: (1) What are the expectations and hopes of the patient and physician, respectively? (2) What are the resources at the disposal of the patient and physician? Obviously, the problem is entirely different if the patient is on a locked ward in a federally financed institution as opposed to seeking outpatient care from a private physician.

It is useful to consider drugs by certain classes as to the extent to which they produce physical dependence, psychological dependence, and tolerance. Table 1 gives an approximate description of this.

Taking the least serious addiction first, tobacco consumption rarely receives active treatment, and little is known about effective forms of treatment other than willpower. It is common among all users to say that they could stop smoking at any time if they really wanted to, but then ignore the factors that lead them to the belief that they do not really want to. Treatment for marihuana smoking is the same as that for tobacco smoking.

The hallucinogen user obtains treatment only when he has undesirable effects of his drug, usually in the form of a state of acute anxiety or hallucinosis. He is usually brought to the physician when psychotherapeutic efforts by his friends in the form of a "talkdown" are ineffective. The safest and most rapidly effective treatment of these conditions is droperidol (Inapsine), 2.5 to 10 mg. intramuscularly or intravenously. Droperidol has the advantage over phenothiazines that there are minimal autonomic side effects; it produces only mild sedation and is of short duration of action in the event that unpleasant extrapyramidal symptoms develop. The person who has continuing flashbacks and anxiety following use of hallucinogens may require prolonged antipsychotic drug treatment or electroconvulsive therapy. We have had one patient refractory to phenothiazines and minor tranquilizers who responded dramatically the second day to lithium carbonate.

Patients get into trouble with stimulants both while "high," when they demonstrate agitation or manic, paranoid, or aggressive behavior, and when they "crash," or have a depression following the prolonged use of stimulants. The

TABLE 1

Types	Physical Dependence	Psychological Dependence	Tolerance
Opiates	++++	++++	++++
Barbiturates and alcohol	++++	++++	++
Amphetamines	+	+++	++++
Cocaine	0	++++	0
Hallucinogens	0	++	+++
Marihuana	0	++	0
Tobacco	0	++	+

treatment of the "high" is the same as the treatment of acute mania, that is, titrating the patient with an antipsychotic drug such as haloperidol, droperidol, or chlorpromazine parenterally. Although the use of a depot preparation such as fluphenazine enanthate will prevent the intense "high" or paranoia resulting from the abuse of stimulants, patients are reluctant to return for treatment since treatment obviates their purpose in getting "high." The "low," depression, or "crash" following a "run" of stimulants is probably the result of depletion of norepinephrine stores in the central nervous system, and these replenish themselves spontaneously in a few days. At this time there is no effective chemical way adequately to effect the process of repletion, and the patient need only be taught that the depression is self-limited. However, a significant number of drug abusers are chronically depressed, and it remains to be tested whether a regular program of antidepressant medication might be therapeutic to some speed users.

Suicide attempts are common among drug users, and occasionally are serious, especially by users of barbiturates or alcohol. Suicidal risk is best evaluated on the basis of general competence of the patient. The better the patient's general reputation for accomplishing what he has said he is going to do, the more likely he is to complete suicide once he starts to consider it. The same impulsive tendencies which give rise to drug abuse cause patients to make frequent suicide attempts, but this is countered by their general incompetence, which often makes these attempts abortive; on balance the suicide rate is high among drug abusers.

Because of the very high rate of relapse after withdrawal from opiates in a hospital, most clinicians now prefer to put opiate addicts on a methadon maintenance program, withdrawing them very slowly on an outpatient basis when they request it and when their life has become sufficiently stable and rewarding that they can live without drugs. We use the following schedule:

For daily doses of methadon over 50 mg., decrease 10 mg per week
then   20-50 mg.,   decrease   5 mg per week
then   8-20 mg.,   decrease   4 mg per week
then   0-8 mg.,   decrease   2 mg per week
then   orange juice for 1 week

Thus, for the average maintenance dose of 100 mg., it will require 5 months to withdraw if everything goes well. Attempts to withdraw more rapidly are usually met with relapse to the previous opiate abused.

Methadon cannot be used for withdrawal from dependence on any other class of drugs except opiates such as heroin, codeine, Percodan, Dilaudid, morphine, and paregoric. Particularly it cannot be used for opiate antagonist analgesics such as pentazocine (Talwyn).

Barbiturates and related drugs such as glutethimide produce physical dependence that may result in fatal convulsions upon abrupt abstinence. Because such addicts usually underestimate their consumption, it is important that the physician treat them with careful observation on a ward and determine their *intoxication threshold*. The intoxication threshold is that amount of pentobarbital required to produce mild intoxication manifested by slurred speech, ataxia, and nystagmus. One starts by giving 0.2 Gm. pentobarbital every 6 hours for 24 hours. If intoxication does not occur within 24 hours, increase the dose to 0.3 Gm. every 6 hours. If no intoxication occurs after another 24 hours, increase to 0.4 Gm. every 6 hours. A very few patients may even have to be raised to 0.4 Gm. every 4 hours. Once intoxication is reached, decrease the dose by 0.1 Gm. every 24 hours until the patient is stabilized. It generally requires a minimum of 1 month's hospitalization to obtain abstinence, and the relapse rate thereafter is exceedingly high.

The major problem in drug dependence is not producing abstinence, it is relapse after "cure." The simplest example is the cigarette smoker who may quit—and relapse—20 times a day. A host of environmental stimuli act as conditioning agents to increase chances for relapse—a neighborhood, certain people, a particular anxiety. As with giving up a fond romance, some persons can avoid relapse by moving to a novel environment. The physiological memory of the drug effect is harder to forget. Many of those who successfully avoid relapse admit that they nevertheless think of drugs daily. It appears that those vulnerable to drug abuse are vulnerable to a host of other impulsive destructive problem-solving maneuvers, and that to improve one, we must attempt to decrease the others simultaneously.

The treatment of the opiate withdrawal state depends upon the facilities available. The opiate abstinence syndrome has never resulted in death and hence is never a medical emergency despite the cries of anguish from the patient. It is perhaps more humane to reduce the amount of opiates gradually, but I suspect that the total amount of discomfort is the same whether one quits abruptly or gradually. Some patients prefer to have the suffering over rapidly, rather than have it drawn out. Unless the patient is on a locked ward, it is futile to attempt withdrawal. Once the patient is under observation, no medication is given until there is objective evidence of withdrawal manifested by piloerection, accompanied by muscle cramps, vomiting, and diarrhea. At that time it is useful to commence methadon, 20 mg. twice a day, and reduce it by 5 mg. per dose until the patient is off in 4 days. The persisting complaints of insomnia are best handled by reassurance that insomnia will be a problem for several months and that the patient had best grow accustomed to it.

It appears that to a large degree, *drugs are people substitutes and vice versa.* A synopsis of the reasoning behind this theory is given by the following four points: (1) people get sick over people; (2) drugs are people substitutes; (3) drug effects are more predictable than people effects; (4) people become necessary to the user only to the extent that they can provide drugs.

All the drug users I have known have been in a state of dis-ease, hurting from their interpersonal relationships at the time the drug dependency started. Such dis-ease may range from the malaise of the poverty-stricken adolescent turning to heroin, to the depression of the middle-aged professional turning to alcohol or sleeping pills, to the unsatisfied drive for achievement of the graduate student user of amphetamines. The drug used and the sociocultural background of the user may be extremely diverse. The drug first used may not be satisfactory, and the person may experiment with a variety of drugs until he either finds one that meets his needs or gives up drug seeking as a way of handling his dis-ease. But when his experience with the drug and the people from whom he obtains drugs help him to allay his discomfort, he is in a position where the probability of his repeating the use of drugs is high. Guilt for utilizing drugs for relief of dis-ease is in part allayed by the gradual development of a paranoid stance which makes him a martyr against those persons who feel that drug use is undesirable. And the *drugs will relieve* his symptoms in a variety of ways, depending on their physiological effects. If he suffers from chronic depression and anticipatory anxiety, he may find that heroin relieves these and provides a feeling of simply not caring in the presence of others. Amphetamines, by relieving fatigue and perhaps occasionally actually improving performance, may provide the ambitious person with actually increased people satisfactions. Although such an improvement is short-lived and gradually leads to deterioration, the memory of what it has done coupled with the fantasy of what it might do becomes more important to the person than the reality of his actual performance. What is most impressive to the drug user is that the drug effect, at least at first, is quite predictable; he can turn himself "on" or "off" at will. It becomes a habitual shortcut for the tedious negotiations necessary to obtain unpredictable people satisfactions. It should not be surprising that with such control over one's feelings, a delusion of omnipotence should gradually appear, for if one can turn oneself on or off, one may in fantasy also turn others on or off. Sometimes this takes the form of apparent altruism in the user giving away drugs to nonusers, in effect controlling them. Coincident with the development of the delusion of omnipotence, there may occur, sometimes for the first time, the development of a conviction about the purpose of life. This new-found purpose in life is simply to obtain drugs and repeat and perpetuate the drug experience.

As this trend develops, people gradually become mere objects to the user, needed only to supply him with drugs. He becomes increasingly condescending and arrogant, even while objectively becoming, paradoxically, most dependent on people and drugs.

Treatment of drug dependency seems to require the provision of equivalent gratification without drugs. Such treatment generally takes the form of an attempt to substitute satisfying people relationships for drug relationships. For the highly addicting drugs this cannot be done while the user continues to take drugs, for the predictability and efficiency of the drugs exceeds that of the people. For this reason, total abstinence is usually essential, with the substitution of satisfying interpersonal relationships during the abstinence period. That this technique is effective for a significant proportion of drug-dependent persons is testified to by the existence of such organizations as Alcoholics Anonymous, Synanon, and Odyssey House.

On the horizon there is hope for much-improved methods of dealing with addiction. It ranges from a more intelligent appreciation by the general public of problems of drugs, to new research developments. The latter include long-acting narcotic antagonists, improved forms of methadon, and aversive conditioning procedures.

SOME RECOMMENDED SOURCE MATERIAL

Books

1. Blachly, P. H. (Ed.): Drug Abuse: Data and Debate. Springfield, Ill., Charles C Thomas, Publisher, 1971.
2. Blachly, P. H.: Seduction: A Conceptual Model in the Drug Dependencies and Other Contagious Social Ills. Springfield, Ill., Charles C Thomas, Publisher, 1971.
3. Interim Report of the Commission of Inquiry into the Non-medical Use of Drugs, Ottawa, Ontario, Canada, 1970.
4. Proceedings of the Third National Conference on Methadon Treatment, New York City, November 14-16, 1970.
5. Report of the Thirty-Third Annual Scientific Meeting of the Committee on Problems of Drug Dependence, Volume I. National Academy of Sciences—National Academy of Engineering, National Research Council, Division of Medical Sciences, Toronto, Ontario, Canada, 1971.
6. Wikler, A. (Ed.): The Addictive States. Baltimore, Williams & Wilkins Co., 1968.
7. Wittenborn, J. R., Smith, J. P., and Wittenborn, S. (Eds.): Communication and Drug Abuse (Proceedings of the Second Rutgers Symposium on Drug Abuse). Springfield, Ill., Charles C Thomas, Publisher, 1970.
8. International Journal of the Addictions.
9. Bulletin on Narcotics, World Health Organization.
10. Journal of Psychedelic Drugs.

Electrosleep Therapy

by Saul H. Rosenthal, M.D.

The term electrosleep is a misnomer as the patient usually does not sleep during the treatment. The term came into use as a direct translation of the Russian term *elektroson,* but whether or not the patient actually falls asleep during the treatments seems irrelevant as far as outcome is concerned.

Electrosleep should be distinguished from "sleep therapy," which usually refers to maintaining a patient in a stuporous state for hours or days by heavy doses of hypnotics. Electrosleep also is not the same as "electroanesthesia," which uses the same kinds of pulsed, positive waves but in a much higher intensity and produces a state of analgesia and immobility. Electrosleep is not related to electroshock therapy in any way and is not the same as subconvulsive electroshock, which uses high-intensity alternating current and usually produces a state of unconsciousness.

Electrosleep as a treatment modality has been developed in Russia and the Soviet bloc countries since 1947. It received great impetus following the publication of a large monograph in 1952 by Giljarowski and Leventsev from the Psychiatric Institute of the Ministry of Public Health of the U.S.S.R.[1] It spread to the Western world in a substantial way following the First and Second International Symposia on Electrosleep and Electroanesthesia, which were held in Graz, Austria, in 1966 and 1969 under the sponsorship of Professor Wageneder from the University of Graz. Our own work at the University of Texas Medical School at San Antonio began in 1969.[2-6]

Background information is available in the Proceedings of the two International Symposia[7,8] and in the *Foreign Science Bulletin* of the United States Library of Congress.[9-12]

Indications for Treatment

At the present time the clearest indications for electrosleep therapy are chronic tension states or chronic anxiety neuroses with or without accompany-

---

Editor's Note: It is the policy of *Current Psychiatric Therapies* to publish all new therapeutic techniques objectively proposed for clinical trial; however, it may be noted that the above study did not employ a control series subjected to placebo procedures such as rapidly vibrating contacts, differential placements of electrodes, etc. Relevant also is the fact that psychiatrists in Czechosolovakia, Bulgaria, and Yugoslavia informed me on a recent tour, that, after prolonged trials, they had found Russian "electrosleep therapy" effective only as a procedure ancillary to suggestive psychotherapy.—J.H.M.

ing reactive depression and chronic insomnia. The best results are probably seen when the anxiety is not clearly related to an acute environmental stress but has persisted chronically with only partial and temporary remissions over a long period of time. As with many other psychiatric treatments, electrosleep therapy works much more effectively in patients with otherwise good ego strength and without serious major personality disorders. As the treatment takes several days, it cannot be used for the immediate management of acute anxiety attacks or hyperventilation syndrome. It may, however, prevent recurrences in chronically anxious patients.

The treatment has proved effective in some patients with chronic primary insomnia unattributable to major anxiety or depressive symptoms. Our results, however, have not been as good with these patients as with those whose insomnia was secondary to chronic anxiety. Our tentative explanation is that patients with chronic insomnia have often had a considerable emotional investment in their insomnia and have built a large part of their lives and identity around it. Electrosleep has no effect at all in our experience on insomnia in the elderly, and for this reason we currently do not attempt to treat patients who are over 62.

The Russians have treated many psychosomatic illnesses that are anxiety related such as bronchial asthma, essential hypertension, and peptic ulcer with electrosleep. We have treated occasional patients with these and other psychosomatic diagnoses in which anxiety obviously played a considerable part and have had encouraging results. We do not, however, have an adequate patient population to be able to make definitive recommendations for treatment of these patient groups. Electrosleep might be tried on an investigational basis as an adjunct in the treatment of anxiety associated with alcoholism or drug addiction. We do not, however, have experience in these areas.

Electrosleep is probably counterindicated in severe endogenous or psychotic depressions or involutional melancholia. We have seen two hospitalized patients with these diagnoses become more agitated with only one or two electrosleep treatments and the treatments have had to be discontinued. Other investigators have shared this experience.

Method

We have customarily given five treatments per week on Monday through Friday. The usual length of a course of treatment is 5 to 15 treatments with our average at present about 10 treatments. Each treatment lasts one-half hour. Treatments are given on an outpatient basis and may be given at any time during the day. The patient requires no special preparation. That is, there is no need for the patient to have an empty stomach or an empty bladder as there is no anesthesia or unconsciousness.

The patient usually reclines in a quiet, semidarkened room or a couch provided with a pillow and sheet. The electrodes, covered by saline-soaked pads, are applied in the sitting position and the cathodes are placed on the closed upper lids, while the anodes are placed behind the mastoid processes. They are held in place firmly but not uncomfortably and should contact as much skin and as little hair as possible. To avoid discomfort, the orbit electrodes should not be in contact with the bridge of the nose and the posterior electrodes should not be touching the ears.

We use a frequency of 100 positive pulses per second and a pulse duration of 1 millisecond with no baseline d.c. bias current. The treatment is begun by slowly increasing the amplitude control and asking the patient to tell the operator when he begins to feel tingling or mild stinging either over the eyes or over the ears. It is usually felt first over the anterior electrodes. Characteristic patient reports include feelings of vibration, itching, slight tingling or stinging, or a feeling of movement or pressure. The current is regulated so that the patient feels a definitely palpable but not uncomfortable sensation. If he reports at any time that the sensation has become uncomfortable, we turn down the amplitude a small amount, which eliminates the uncomfortable sensation. Our treatment current is usually in the range of 0.5 to 1.5 milliamps. The readings on the dials of the various commercially manufactured machines may be inaccurate, but this has not caused a problem as we regulate the current according to the patient's perception rather than the dial reading. Someone should be with the patient at all times during the treatment in case the patient should become frightened or have an uncomfortable increase in sensation.

If the patient falls asleep during the treatment, at the end of the half-hour treatment he is awakened. The patients feel no confusion, memory loss, or disorientation although they may report that they feel sedated and desire to sleep following the treatment.

Response to Treatment

The patient is usually mildly apprehensive before the first treatment, but his apprehension will decrease with partial relaxation. The next day the patient will report that following the first treatment he felt sedated and perhaps took a nap in the afternoon. He may feel some relaxation and report sleeping more soundly at night. During the second and third treatments he is more likely to relax during the treatment, drifting into a twilight sleep or dozing. Following the second and third treatments, the patient may or may not feel as sedated during the afternoon but may feel more elevation of mood for several hours following the treatment. Anxiety may be decreased, and some increase in libido is occasionally reported. Sleep improves but most patients report an increase in dreaming. By the fourth or fifth day the patient may report an increase in energy and alertness during the day. Both sedation and mild euphoric effects following the treatment are no longer as prominent. Anxiety may be reported as decreased and improvement of sleep maintained. The remission of symptoms has been maintained for variable times ranging from one week to one year.

Side Effects. Blurring of vision for 5 or 10 minutes following the removal of the electrodes has been reported almost universally. This is ascribed to the pressure of the anterior electrodes on the eyes as it is observed whether or not there is any application of electrical current. Occasionally patients report a mild headache following treatments lasting several hours, and usually relieved by aspirin. Some patients find the increase in dreaming uncomfortable.

Although the treatment is relatively new in the United States and there have been no long-term follow-up studies, there have been over 20 years of experience in the Soviet bloc countries which seem to indicate a remarkable absence of serious side effects. Electrosleep may indeed have fewer side effects than most of the medications currently in use and certainly has fewer obvious CNS side effects than electroshock therapy.

As a substitute for medication, electrosleep has several advantages. It is possibly more effective. It avoids the common medication side effects as well as problems of medication abuse, incorrect dosage, and suicidal and accidental overdoses.

REFERENCES

1. Giljarowski, W. A., and Leventsev, N. M.: Electrosleep. Berlin, Veb Verlag Volk und Gesundheit, 1956.
2. Rosenthal, S. H., and Wulfsohn, N. L.: Studies of Electrosleep with Active and Simulated Treatment. Curr. Ther. Res. 12(3):126-130, (March) 1970.
3. Rosenthal, S. H., and Wulfsohn, N. L.: Electrosleep: A Preliminary Communication. J. Nerv. Ment. Dis. 151(3):146-151, 1970.
4. Rosenthal, S. H., and Wulfsohn, N. L.: Electrosleep—A Clinical Trial. Amer. J. Psychiat 127(4):175-176 (October) 1970.
5. Rosenthal, S. H., and Calvert, L. F.: Electrosleep: Personal Subjective Experiences. Biol. Psychiat. (in press).
6. Rosenthal, S. H.: Electrosleep: A Double-Blind Clinical Study. Biol. Psychiat. (in press).
7. Wageneder, F. M., and St. Schuy, G.: Electrotherapeutic Sleep and Electroanaesthesia. Proceedings of the First International Symposium, Graz, Austria, September. New York, Excerpta Medica, 1966.
8. Wageneder, F. M., and St. Schuy, G.: Electrotherapeutic Sleep and Electroanaesthesia. Proceedings of the Second International Symposium, Graz, Austria, September, Amsterdam, Excerpta Medica, 1970.
9. Dodge, C.: Electrosleep, Electroanesthesia, and Electroneural Diagnostics and Therapeutics. For. Sci. Bull. 3(3):46-64, 1967.
10. Iwanovsky, A., and Dodge, C. H.: Electrosleep and Electroanesthesia—Theory and Clinical Experience. For. Sci. Bull. 4(2):1-64, 1968.
11. Iwanovsky, A.: Report of International Progress in Cerebral Electrotherapy (Electrosleep) and Electroanesthesia. For. Sci. Bull. 5(10):15-40 (October) 1969.
12. Wageneder, F. M., Iwanovsky, A., and Dodge, C. H.: Electrosleep (Cerebral Electrotherapy) and Electroanesthesia—The International Effort at Evaluation. For. Sci. Bull. 5(4):1-104, 1969.

PART IV

FAMILY THERAPY

Genetic Counseling

by Henry T. Lynch, M.D., and William L. Harlan, M.D.

It has been estimated that diseases of clearly defined genetic origin now comprise about 6 percent of the admissions to pediatric hospitals, and another 15 percent of these admissions are for causes of less well-defined genetic content. In addition, genetic disorders account for a major fraction of pediatric deaths. In the case of adults this number undoubtedly increases remarkably when one considers the role of genetics in some of the leading killers of man: e.g., diabetes mellitus, certain forms of cancer, a large number of progressively deteriorating neurologic disorders, and heart disease including generalized arteriosclerosis.

Developments in the field of medical genetics have been almost explosive since the turn of the century, heralded initially by the rediscovery of Mendel's genetic principles and followed by the stimulus of such brilliant investigators as Garrod and Galton in England, Dahlberg in Denmark, Verschuer and Weinberg in Germany, and Oliver, Stern, Kallmann, and others in the United States. Genetic fundamentals provided by these scientists have now been cast in new perspective through the development of molecular concepts. There are now amazing insights into the "stuff of genetics," namely DNA, through the work of the Nobel laureates Watson and Krick, through the specific gene-enzyme and related biochemical concepts of Tatum, Beadle, and many others, and through the developments in human cytogenetics beginning in the 1950s. Thus, our newly emerged medical genetic discipline has been founded with sound mathematical and statistical expertise and significantly abetted by biochemical, physiological, and cytologic sciences, all of which have been recently adapted and nurtured by physicians.[1] The development and application of mass screening methods for many types of genetic diseases foster their early recognition, so that substantial benefit may be achieved through early counseling and therapy.[2]

Many physicians who were graduated from medical school 10 or more years ago have had little exposure to genetics. Even recent graduates whose grounding in genetics has been necessarily brief in an already crowded curriculum must find it quite difficult to keep abreast of recent developments in this rapidly expanding field. The result is that physicians sometimes refer their cases for counseling to nonmedically trained geneticists at colleges and universities. But the genetic counselor should first of all be a physician, whose perspective differs from that of nonmedically trained geneticists who frequently place emphasis only on the patient's request for factual information concerning the inheritance of a particular disease. Such a counselor is not sufficiently informed about matters of pathogenesis, treatment, and prognosis; therefore, he must necessarily limit his discussion to those areas in which he is competent, namely, the matter of genetic mechanisms and risk factors. This approach is sufficient when the medical problem at hand involves only a small amount of significant feeling content, such as the genetics of eye color, hair color, or blood type; however, when it involves diseases which carry significant morbidity and/or mortality, a cursory and superficial approach to the problem will not suffice. The counselor must have an awareness of the emotions, feelings, and attitudes of the person he is counseling as well as those of other members of the family who may be involved. Furthermore, he must be alert to the dynamic interactions taking place within the family milieu and must bring to bear all his skill and experience in case management in order to allay unfounded fears, dispel doubts, and generally assist the patient and his family to understand the disease in question and their relationship to it in a true and reasonable perspective.[3-5]

Technique of Genetic Counseling

If the proband is the informant and the person seeking help, counseling may closely approximate individual supportive therapy. In addition to the history, a detailed physical examination searching for subtle clinical manifestations and minimal stigmata of the disease as well as unrelated pathology should be performend.

When appropriate one may express an interest in examining other members of the family. The patient's participation in achieving this is to be encouraged, since both patient and counselor often obtain additional insights with regard to the emotional impact of the disease on the family. Often one will discover additional cases in the family, or one may detect undiscovered minimally affected *forme fruste* cases when one is allowed to examine supposedly unaffected family members. As better methods of treatment of genetic conditions are developed, the importance of early recognition of such cases is self-evident.

In a second situation the person seeking genetic counseling may not be the proband and may or may not be at risk for the disease. In such instances the physician should carefully appraise the goals and the degree of ego involvement his patient has with the carrier of the disease. For example, he may be a close personal friend, or he may have married into a family in which a hereditary disorder has been manifested; he may have one or more affected children; or he, himself, may have minimal, moderate, or severe manifestations of the particular hereditary defect. An appreciation of the physical and mental limitations imposed by the particular disease is also important, for all these factors will determine the overall potential of the patient in terms of occupation, marriage, and future goals. An example follows:

Case Report: Huntington's Chorea[6]

The proband was a physician who had been in general practice. He had an insidious onset of neurologic and psychiatric manifestations of Huntington's chorea beginning in his early forties with progression to a moderately advanced degree. His 26-year-old son, a senior medical student, was laboring under severe apprehension as to whether he might eventually show manifestations of this genetic disorder. Since there is no way of detecting the carrier state of this disease, save for the demonstration of clinical signs, his anxiety was increased because of his knowledge and study of the affliction, the presence of which in his family he had not known until after he was married and his wife was already pregnant. The son stated: "We would never have had a child [now age three] had we known about the disease in the family."

Any discussion of the possibility of detecting this disease at the subclinical level in this patient met with considerable anguish. He finally blurted out: "I would never want to be tested for the presence of this disease should a test ever become available. I think if I found out that I was affected, I would commit suicide." The patient's brother, an engineer, expressed a similar reaction.

Interviews with other members of the family showed fear and, in some cases, rejection of affected members by unaffected relatives. For example, in an attempt to elicit cooperation from an unaffected sister of the proband we were told that the less she knew about the disease the better and that she did not want to have anything to do with relatives who were affected. Nevertheless, empathetic listening did provide several of the relatives with the opportunity to appraise the problem objectively. In the case of the proband's physician-son, he and his wife are now contemplating adoption and seem to have achieved some insight into their problem. It is apparent that a recital of genetic risk information to relatives in the above family would be without merit. The counselor would require not only a detailed knowledge of the natural history of this disease but also sufficient understanding of the emotional pressures existent in the family. The art of genetic counseling rests in being able to temper comments about genetic risk factors not only with the necessary accuracy but also in a manner which embodies a full empathetic appreciation of the emotional content.

Discussion

The presence of hereditary diseases in a kindred often produces severe anxiety hostility, and misdirected guilt in both affected and nonaffected family members.[1,7-9] Feelings of "punishment" are sometimes noted. Reproductive performance may be curtailed.[1,7] Affected members may make extraordinary efforts to conceal developing symptoms, thus avoiding detection and therapy.[10]

Emotional responses to "genetic factors" may in part be conditioned by bizarre concepts of inheritance.[11] In order to be effective, genetic counseling must be predicated upon the fact that there is often confusion and bewilderment concerning the presence of "hereditary" disease in the family. Unfortunately, members of the community in which the family resides may also react to hereditary disorders with similar misconceptions. Hence, depending upon the particular sequelae, a family with hereditary disease may be affected by both intrafamilial strife as well as community "scapegoating" and ostracism.[12] Krush and associates[12] found numerous emotional ramifications in a family with a grotesquely disfiguring hereditary disease (mandibulofacial dysostosis). The impact of this disease was demonstrated from the standpoints of community, kindred, and interfamilial reactions. A vicious cycle existed so that the family was disparaged for the grotesque "fishmouth" facies of affected individuals, severely handicapping them in education and occupation.

In counseling over one thousand families with hereditary diseases,[1,7-9] it has become apparent that family members are far less interested in the esoteric aspects of mendelian ratios and empiric risk figures than in the conflicts occasioned by the presence of hereditary disease in the family. Needed most at this time is a compassionate physician who is willing to provide an empathetic "listening ear."[8] This may take several sessions, but it is only after the emotional content has been expressed and accepted that the basic biological issues and modes of inheritance may be presented to the patient.

A useful approach to this aspect of counseling has been to teach methods of pedigree construction to mature family members. They are then taught to incorporate the names of individuals known to be affected into the format of the pedigree. This encourages active participation by family members and enables them to comprehend the manner of transmission of the disease in their family.

Early Hereditary Deaths. Bird et al.[13] investigated a large kindred afflicted with hereditary telangiectasia with early deaths. Attitudes of family members seemed to reflect an increased interest in the importance of family traditions and values on the one hand, but with a diminished interest in the importance of the individual per se on the other. The family was drawn together and became rather clannish as a result of the deaths of their members; interestingly, defensive denials were prominent, and fecundity was increased.

A family with chronic interstitial nephritis[14] and one with Lindau's disease,[15] both showing early deaths from these hereditary diseases, were similarly studied. Denial and repression were again prominent but interest in the family did not overshadow that in the individual, nor was fecundity emphasized.

Interview material which we obtained on two families with autosomal recessive diseases (i.e., cystinosis and transposition of the great vessels) with hereditary deaths in children has shown striking similarities with respect to underlying psychodynamics.[8] In both families, reproductive performance ceased—by surgical sterilization in one and diligent use of contraceptive techniques in the other. Furthermore, the curtailment of reproduction was not limited to the parents of the affected progeny, but rather had been manifested throughout the family.[7,8,16]

Family Orientation[1,7-17]

Emphasis upon the family as a unit in general medicine and psychiatry is by no means a new concept.[17] Certainly in dealing with a hereditary disease wherein the proband shares a varying quantity of genes with blood relatives, it is only logical and practical that the family be viewed as a functioning and therapeutically concerned unit. For example, when decisions are made between husband and wife concerning taking a "chance" on another pregnancy, the physician-counselor should not focus his entire attention upon just one of the marital partners without bringing the other spouse into the issue with full recognition of his or her role, feelings, attitudes, identifications, and responsibility for future progeny. In general, the more significant the particular genetic trait is from the standpoint of such factors as cosmetically disfiguring diseases, psychiatric aberrations, early childhood deaths, or chronic and progressively debilitating diseases, the more disturbed the family unit may become,[1] and the greater the necessity for achieving homeostasis within the family.[6,7,16].

Genetic Counseling in Psychiatry

Not only in private psychiatry but also within the state mental hospital setting the opportunities for the use of genetic counseling are many and varied. With the development of new policies in state mental health departments directed toward outpatient treatment of mental illness, keeping the patient out of the hospital and functioning optimally close to his home there are developing ancillary services, among them genetic counseling. We submit that the effectiveness of such clinics will depend at least in part on adequate educational programs in genetics and genetic counseling as a part of psychiatric residency training, together with continued independent interest on the part of practicing psychiatrists in this newly emerging aspect of medical practice.

REFERENCES

1. Lynch, H. T.: Dynamic Genetic Counseling for Clinicians. Springfield, Ill., Charles C Thomas, Publisher, 1969, p. 354.
2. Clow, C. L., Reade, T. M., and Scriver, C. R.: Management of Hereditary Metabolic Disease: The Role of Allied Health Personnel. New Eng. J. Med. 284:1292-1298 (June) 1971.

3. McKusick, V. A.: Mendelian Inheritance in Man: Catalogs of Autosomal Dominant, Autosomal Recessive and X-Linked Phenotypes, 2nd ed. Baltimore, The Johns Hopkins Press, 1968, pp. 54.

4. Kaplan, A. R.: The Genetics of Schizophrenia. Springfield, Ill., Charles C Thomas, Publisher, 1971 (in press).

5. Goodman, R. M.: Genetic Disorders of Man. Boston, Little, Brown & Company, 1970, pp. 1009.

6. Lynch, H. T., Harlan, W. L., and Dyhrberg, J.: Subjective Perspective of Genetic Counseling: Huntington's Chorea. Arch. Gen. Psychiat. (Chicago) 1971 (in press).

7. Tips, R. L., Smith, G. S., Lynch, H. T., and McNutt, C. W.: The "Whole Family" Concept in Clinical Genetics. Amer. J. Dis. Child. 107:67-76 (January) 1964.

8. Lynch, H. T., Krush, T. P., Krush, A. J., and Tips, R. L.: Psychodynamics of Early Hereditary Deaths: Role of the Medical Genetics Counselor. Amer. J. Dis. Child. 108:605-610 (December) 1964.

9. Lynch, H. T., Tips, R. L., and Krush, A. J.: Psychodynamics in a Chronic Debilitating Hereditary Disease: Myotonia Dystrophica. Arch. Gen. Psychiat. 14:154-157, 1966.

10. Krush, A. J., Lynch, H. T., and Magnuson, C. W.: Attitudes Toward Cancer in a "Cancer Family": Implications for Cancer Detection. Amer. J. Med. Sci. 249:432-438 (April) 1965.

11. Glenister, T. W.: Fantasies, Facts and Foetuses: The Interplay of Fancy and Reason in Teratology. Med. Hist. 8:15-30 (January) 1964.

12. Krush, A., Krush, T. P., and Lynch, H. T.: Psycho-social Factors in a Family with a Disfiguring Genetic Fault. Psychosomatics 16:391-396, 1965.

13. Bird, R. M., Hammarsten, J. F., Marshall, R. A., and Robinson, R. R.: A Family Reunion: A Study of Hereditary Hemorrhagic Telangiectasia, New Eng. J. Med. 257:105-109, 1957.

14. Langsley, D. G.: Psychology of a Doomed Family. Amer. J. Psychother. 15:531-538, 1961.

15. Langsley, D. G., Wolton, R. V., and Goodman, T. A.: Family with Hereditary Fatal Disease. Arch. Gen. Psychiat. (Chicago) 10:647-652, 1964.

16. Tips, R. L., and Lynch, H. T.: Impact of Genetic Counseling upon Family Milieu. J.A.M.A. 185:183-186, 1963.

17. Sholevar, G.: Family Therapy. J. Albert Einstein Med. Ctr. 13:61-66, 1970.

Psychiatric Therapy of Marital Problems: Modern Techniques*

by Bernard L. Greene, M.D.

No one current model can describe the transactions within a marriage. All behavior has meaning, and all individuals are motivated by internal activities. In addition to this *intrapersonal system,* every individual has meaningful relationships with others (*interpersonal system*) and lives in a sociocultural matrix (*environmental system*). Marital problems results from these three systems continually transacting with each other and creating permutations which are dysfunctional.

Von Bertalanffy defines a system as a complex of components in mutual interaction. He postulates open systems that have their own inherent lawfulness. Each system consists of transacting elements within penetrable boundaries, thus ensuring "openness." Each system has a temporal and spatial existence with structure derived from its past; its present is relatively stable; and its future has possible evolutionary potential. Each system maintains its organization by goal-seeking activities characterized by "equifinality," indicating that the same final state can be reached from different initial conditions and in different ways. Each system may maintain itself by realigning gradients, by partially sacrificing structure or function, or by decreasing its boundaries to permeability. Finally, each system is in active interplay with other systems in its environment which are significant for its viability. Thus the focus in evaluating a marital problem is directed to its relationship to general systems theory (GST).

Since management of a marital problem begins with the first evaluative session, it is important that the therapist do something within the first 10 minutes of the initial interview to alleviate anxiety and/or hostility in order to establish a "working alliance" with the patient. An early appointment is advisable, as marital crises respond best when dealt with at the height of tension. The request for help may be unilateral or bilateral. At one extreme are those who are adamant that they are not in need of help and the problem is entirely due to their mate. At the other end are those couples who are willing to do anything to alleviate the marital discord and who are eager for counsel. Often a

---

*The material in this chapter appeared in somewhat different form in *A Clinical Approach to Marital Problems: Evaluation and Management,* by Bernard L. Greene, Springfield, Ill., Charles C Thomas, Publisher, 1970. Courtesy of the publisher.

spouse will refuse to be interviewed. The therapist should take the initiative and telephone the partner, explaining that his information would be most valuable in dealing with his spouse's complaints. Infrequently (5 percent) will a partner refuse to be interviewed.

The stage is set for therapy on a transactional basis at the time of the first request for an appointment. With the expectation that both partners participate in the initial evaluations, they usually do. Focusing on the *marriage* as the "patient" with a clearly stated rationale strongly influences the expectations and approach of the therapist and the partners. The evaluation consists of one to three individual sessions (usually two), plus a final conjoint diagnostic and disposition (CDD) session where the transactions between the spouses can be observed firsthand. They are told that a statement will be made at the CDD as to impressions and recommendations.

The individual diagnostic phase permits each spouse fully to relate his presenting complaints. Being seen individually permits revealing so-called "family secrets," e.g., infidelity, and expression of feelings in their full flower without fear of retaliation from the partner. Conjoint interviews are indicated from the first session on when the psychiatrist senses that individual sessions will call forth distortion or paranoid reactions.

At the end of the first individual interview, the patient is given two biographical marital questionnaires (BMQ), one for each of the partners, and told that the BMQs hasten the evaluation if completed and mailed in before the next interview. Data from the BMQs have proved useful in obtaining background information on the spouses, sometimes being obtained more readily than in the individual session. The therapist should be exposed to a conceptual frame that permits a broad coverage of many potentially significant factors. In any couple only some of these factors may be of immediate concern, e.g., vasectomy.

Biographical Marital Questionnaire
(Personal Data and Source of Referral)

What are your specific complaints about your marriage? First circle and then describe:

    a. Lack of communication
    b. Constant arguments
    c. Unfilled emotional needs
    d. Sexual dissatisfaction
    e. Financial disagreements
    f. In-law trouble
    g. Infidelity
    h. Conflicts about children
    i. Domineering spouse
    j. Suspicious spouse
    k. Others

Why are you *now* seeking help?

If you have received any help with respect to your marriage, circle the following: psychiatrist, psychologist, physician, clergy, social worker, counselor, agency, other. Name of person and date. Give your opinion of the results.

Have *you* or *your spouse* ever attempted suicide? If so, give details.

The getting-married phase: How did you meet your spouse?

Describe your courtship, giving duration and whether smooth, stormy, etc.

Did you have a honeymoon? Describe your reactions, partner's behavior, etc.

Any previous marriages? If yes, did the marriages end by divorce, death, or desertion? Give details.

Original family:
Father: name, occupation, age if living, age at death.

Mother: name, occupation, age if living, age at death.
Brothers and sisters: First name only, age, sex.

Describe your parents, what they were like as people, and how they got along in their marriage. How did you get along with them? Describe your family's circumstances as you were growing up. Include anything else that would give a clearer picture of your family experiences and relationships.

Relationship with your children: Describe your children and your relationship with them. What are the problems and conflicts that arise, and how do you deal with them? How do you feel about being a parent?

Describe the kind of person you are: feelings of inferiority, sensitivity, anxiety, etc.

School adjustment: How well did you do as far as grades were concerned? What extracurricular activities did you participate in? What problems did you have in school?

Medical history: Family physician, name, and address.

What is your present state of health?

When did you have your last medical checkup?

What serious medical illnesses have you had and when?

What surgical operations have you had and when?

What drugs are you presently taking?

How much do you smoke?

How much do you drink and how often?

Do you think you drink too much?

Describe your participation in social and civic activities. What are your personal hobbies and interests? How much satisfaction do you get from these activities? What problems do you have in this area?

Describe your job or occupation. Describe your feelings about your work. How do you get along with your coworkers and employer? Have you changed jobs frequently? If so, give details.

Religion: What is your religious preference? What religious and other church-sponsored activities do you participate in? How often is your participation? How have the teachings and values of your church and your faith influenced your marriage?

Any additional comments you wish to make about your marriage?

The routine CDD is the end point of the evaluative phase. After the individual sessions with each couple, unless conjoint sessions were begun at the outset, the couple is seen together for both diagnostic and planning purposes. The therapist must continually be on the alert as to the varied ways marital problems may masquerade or be expressed in vocational ineffectiveness, alcoholism, and so on. As one describes a person's needs and motivations, the implication is often made that these patterns of behavior are pathological per se. Thus it is easy to talk of a man's need to be mothered, or of his need to dominate. But none of these needs is necessarily pathological, and many are worthwhile. In evaluating a marriage, we observe whether the husband wants to be mastered whereas his wife likes to dominate. This does not mean that the marriage is conflictual in that area. What is important is the totality of the transactions between the couple and not to condemn overtly or covertly such transactions in psychological terms. The therapist has the responsibility of performing diagnostic duties and reaching a decision before he begins therapeutic action.

There is as yet no generally accepted classification of marital disharmony. In keeping with the general system theory, all three systems are considered in marital diagnosis. Otto Pollak's observations on the marriage cycle are valuable in understanding the dynamics of marital diagnosis. He has described how a marriage may be disturbed by failure of need complementarity between the spouses in the areas of interpersonal reorientation, sexuality, finances, and ego strengthening as the family passes from one developmental phase to another. Dicks's concepts of projective identification and unconscious collusion are also helpful in arriving at a marital diagnosis. Further, communicational clarification, involving the interpersonal system particularly, is of value. Marital games analysis (Bernean) adds a valuable parameter in understanding the marital dynamics.

Therapies

The complexity of our society results in great variations in marital patterns and greater flexibility in therapeutic techniques. Clinical necessity, therapeutic failures, and advancing knowledge require further flexibility in technique. The therapist must evaluate the problem of each couple and decide intuitively what technique or combination of techniques is most applicable at any particular moment. I have proposed a "six-C" classification of therapeutic modalities.

I. Supportive therapy.
   A. *Crisis counseling.*
II. Intensive therapy.
   A. *Classical psychoanalytic psychotherapy.*
   B. *Collaborative therapy.*
   C. *Concurrent therapy.*
   D. *Conjoint marital therapy.*
   E. *Combined therapies:*
      1. Simple.
      2. Conjoint *family* therapy.
      3. Combined-collaborative therapy.
      4. Marital group psychotherapy.

In the evolution of therapeutic techniques, I began by focusing upon the individual, on the dyadic one-to-one relationship. Treatment failures necessitated the inclusion of the transactions between husband and wife as well as their personalities. The triadic approaches, including concurrent, conjoint marital, and combined techniques, were thus utilized. Finally, because of therapeutic impasses I had to include children, in the clinical setting, who were contributing to the marital discord through scapegoating or other roles. Treatment can thus be visualized in terms of a spectrum of therapeutic settings, with the dyadic approaches of classical and collaborative techniques at one end, the triadic approaches of concurrent, conjoint marital, and combined therapies in the middle, and conjoint family therapy and marital group therapy at the other end.

The principles of management of marital discord include: mutual responsibility not only for the discord but also for its solution; a review of the marriage contract after Don D. Jackson; a target date of about 12 sessions—usually a therapeutic trial of 3 months with an "open-door" policy; a nuclear dynamic model of the family; the use of the transient structured distance (TSD) where indicated; the use of therapeutic principles in keeping with the GST; and the importance of confidentiality. I stress that *the patient is the marriage.* I specifically emphasize that past behavior furnishes a historical perspective but that each spouse will be responsible for current behavior. The contract I present is a biased one, later to be changed if mutually acceptable to the spouses. In many couples where infidelity was a major source of conflict, the stress on exclusiveness in the marital contract often alleviates anxiety and hastens the therapeutic process.

The nuclear dynamic model is presented to the couple in terms of the possible outcome of their marriage. This model can be visualized as a circle containing an enclosed smaller circle and thus having an internal and external boundary. Four stages occur in the progressive dissolution of a marriage; i.e., in a durable incompatible marriage both internal and external boundaries are intact; emotional divorce occurs where the internal boundary is disrupted; separation disrupts the internal boundary and fragments the external boundary; and in divorce both external and internal boundaries are disrupted.

TSD delineates rules and roles in certain couples with marital problems. This distancing maneuver may be structured either at the beginning or during the therapeutic process and has been found to be both diagnostic and therapeutic. The rules are based on conflict areas. In three-fifths of the couples where the TSD was introduced, one or both spouses had reached the conclusion that separation or divorce was inevitable. As a diagnostic tool, the TSD is used to clarify the status of the marriage, to determine the readiness of a spouse for separation, and so on. As a therapeutic tool, it can be used to neutralize pyramiding hostility and/or anxiety that threatens to prematurely disrupt the marriage.

Two therapeutic principles in keeping with GST should be kept in mind:

1. It is impossible to alter significantly one element in any of the three systems without producing changes in the entire system.
2. It is futile to select one element for attention and action while ignoring and disregarding the others.

The therapist must be able to adapt his therapeutic approach to the couple's individual, as well as mutual, needs—*tailored crisis counseling:* an orientation stressing sociocultural forces and explicitly acknowledging the implications of the "here-and-now" situation. The counseling approaches were used in 38 percent of a total of over a thousand couples treated in the last 35 years. Since the indications and contraindications for the various techniques are the same in counseling and in intensive therapy, each treatment modality will be presented separately.

The classic approach can be defined as a dyadic one-to-one relationship between the therapist and his patient. In this type of treatment the therapists of each spouse do not communicate. Thus confidentiality of all transactions between the therapist and patient is crucial. The classic approach was used in about 10 percent of the couples receiving counseling or intensive psychotherapy. In the classic approach therapy is focused on the individual's psychodynamics with the marriage as the backdrop. How patterns of behavior develop receives selective focus over how spouses react to these patterns.

The indications for the classic approach include:

1. Therapist's knowledge of acting-out behavior ("family secrets") by one partner of which the other is unaware, e.g., continuous infidelity or homosexuality.
2. Personal preference of one or both spouses.
3. Immaturity in a spouse which precludes sharing the therapist.
4. Conviction in one spouse that he or she has to figure out his own way irrespective of the consequences to his partner.
5. When spouses have widely differing goals in terms of the marriage problem.

The contraindication to the classic approach is when a spouse has moderate to severe paranoid reactions to being "told on" or being influenced by the other spouse. This suspicious behavior by a spouse leads to repeated questioning as to what went on in the partner's individual session and frequent distortion.

In the collaborative approach, both spouses are treated individually but currently by separate therapists who communicate with the knowledge and permission of each partner. The collaborative approach, a dyadic one-to-one relationship, was used in about 10 percent of the couples receiving counseling or intensive psychotherapy. Martin and Bird were pioneers in 1948 in the development of this technique. To be effective this approach requires *regular scheduled meetings* between the therapists.

The following are the indications for this approach:

1. Opposition of one spouse to being treated by the same therapist as his partner.
2. Initial hostility of one spouse toward the therapist.
3. Referral from another therapist because of his personal reasons, e.g., discomfort in the triadic setting.
4. Referral from another therapist because the partner has created therapeutic complications.

The contraindications for the collaborative technique are the same as for the classic approach.

Experience has shown difficulties of communication between therapists with this technique. Mutual trust and confidence does not prevent cross-transference difficulties between the therapists. Most important in this technique is the loss of the strategical center for integrating all revelant observations of the marriage, when the events and perceptions are parceled out between therapists.

In the concurrent approach, both spouses are treated individually but synchronously by the same therapist. This triadic technique is of value when a therapy must deal with elements of the intrapersonal system and with the family transactions as well. Mittlemann pioneered in the use of this technique in 1948.

The concurrent approach was used in about 25 percent of the couples in counseling and the couples receiving intensive therapy.

The indications for this approach include:

1. When the mental status of one spouse has overwhelmed his partner.
2. When insight into behavior patterns as they affect each partner is needed to produce changes in behavior.
3. When counseling procedures have indicated that one or both spouses could profit from a deeper understanding of the components of their three systems.

The contraindications for this approach are:

1. Severe psychoses or severe character disorders.
2. Paranoid reactions.
3. Suspicious attitudes toward the communications of spouses.
4. Excessive sibling-rivalry attitudes.
5. "Family secrets."
6. Very rigid defenses which, if broken, might produce a severe psychoneurosis, a psychosomatic crisis, or a psychosis.

In the conjoint marital approach both partners are seen together by the same therapist in the same session. This technique was used in 44 percent of the couples in counseling and 16 percent in intensive therapy.

The indications for this approach include:

1. Therapeutic impasse with the concurrent approach.
2. Paranoid or suspicious behavior of one spouse.
3. Economics—the cost of treatment is halved.
4. When explosiveness of the marital situation demands speed in bringing order to the family environment.
5. Need to foster communication between the partners.
6. To point out not merely the differences but the possibility of complementation in the transactions between the couple.

The contraindications for conjoint therapy are the same as in the concurrent approach.

In indicated couples seeing both partners jointly provided more access to the marital dynamics. Conjoint sessions give the advantage of heightened perception. Direct observation facilitates more objective evaluation of the partners' behavior and limits the need to judge distortion from more indirect data. With both partners in the session, the therapist can observe the positive strivings and values of the marriage. An important advantage is the opportunity afforded the partners via the therapist to receive a lesson in how to communicate. In conjoint sessions, a couple can work out reality problems which they have not been able to solve at home.

In the combined approaches in marital disharmony, the couple is seen in a variety of dyadic and triadic clinical settings:

1. Simple: a combination of individual, concurrent, and conjoint sessions in various purposeful combinations.

2. Conjoint family therapy in which one or more of the children are included in the therapeutic setting.

3. Combined-collaborative, in which each spouse is treated individually by separate therapists and all four persons meet together at regular intervals.

4. Marital group therapy: ideally, four couples are seen with one or two therapists.

The variability in marital patterns and the unpredictable therapeutic course necessitated the technical variations found in the combined approaches. The treatment process in the combined techniques is based on a plan of active support, including environmental manipulation, complementary goals, clarification of role expectations and enactments, redirection of intrapersonal energies, and evocation of "healthier" communication. A combined approach differs in many ways from the techniques previously described. When the dyadic and triadic sessions are combined, the interview takes on different meanings for all the participants.

When four out of five marriages are having various degrees of marital disharmony, with many ending in separation or divorce, it becomes the responsibility of the therapist to be in the forefront of prevention. There are three areas of prevention: primary, secondary, and tertiary. Primary prevention attempts to eradicate marital problems in three areas:

1. Premarital counseling.
2. Marital counseling—the "well-marriage unit."
3. Remarital counseling.

The "well-marriage unit" is similar in philosophy to the well-baby clinic. Currently I recommend a periodic marital checkup after premarital or remarital counseling, yearly after marriage for three visits, then every 3 years for three visits, and then once every 5 years. Secondary prevention in marriage attempts to recognize and treat a marital crisis at the earliest possible time so as to reduce the length or severity of the problem. Tertiary prevention either attempts to minimize the repercussions to a request for a divorce or consists of divorce counseling per se. In divorce or remarital counseling, frequently the same forces are present, and any one or combination of the following situations obtain:

1. Mourning process by a spouse.
2. When the spouse is still a "phallic symbol" to the partner and reacts with panic or severe anxiety.
3. Rage reactions toward spouse due to rejection, to separation from the children, or to protracted legal transactions and/or terms of the separation.

Institutional Family Therapy*

by Gene M. Abroms, M.D.

Since hospitalizing anyone at all, much less his family, runs contrary to many trends in the philosophy, if not the actual practice, of contemporary psychiatric care, I propose to review some of the applications and apparent benefits of this approach,[1] in an effort not to replace one fad with another but to arrive at some precise indications for this form of treatment.

Characteristics of the Patients

The milieu therapy units (two 21-bed wards) of the University of Wisconsin Hospitals preferentially select patients with early acute psychiatric disorders, of whom approximately 15 percent are University students. The first 100 initial patients with whom additional family members were admitted were from 17 to 64 years old, with concentration in the 18-30 range; there were 32 diagnoses of schizophrenia, 24 of affective psychosis, 23 of personality disorder, 16 of neurosis, and 5 of miscellaneous disorders. The 672 nonfamily index cases admitted during the same period (March, 1968, to July, 1969) had a similar diagnostic breakdown. During the treatment of these 100 index patients, 126 additional family members, mostly marital partners (45 husbands, 26 wives), ranging in age from 2 months to 68 years, entered the hospital. On 15 occasions both parents of the initial patient came in; on 7 occasions one or more children were admitted; and in 4 cases both parents plus siblings and in 3 cases a spouse with children were admitted. Fifty-one percent of the additional family members were diagnosed as having personality disorders; 9 percent neurotic disorders; 6 percent schizophrenia; and 4 percent miscellaneous disorders, leaving only 30 percent who were judged not to warrant individual psychopathological diagnoses.

The Program

In referring to "family therapy" we mean nothing more than the psychiatric treatment of two or more members of a nuclear family as an ongoing group. Within a therapeutic milieu such as ours, several therapists always work collaboratively with each family. Typically, a resident psychiatrist and one or

---

*Adapted by permission from Amer. J. Psychiat. 127:1363-1370, 1971.

two members of the nursing and nursing aid staff are involved, but a supervising psychiatrist, social worker, or other professional may sit in from time to time.

We began family treatment by taking mothers with postpartum reactions and their babies into the hospital, with the idea of treating the mother's symptoms and teaching her the requisite homemaking and child-care skills involved in raising an infant. This type of work, however, does not commit the treatment team to a specific family-dynamic model, as was evident from our initial individual-dynamic emphasis. We were forced to bridge this theoretical gap when we began admitting both parents of psychotic young adults. Our first case was typical in many respects.

Case 1. The initial patient had been confined in a well-known psychiatric hospital for the previous three years where, after individual therapy, drugs, and electroconvulsive therapy (ECT), she was still bizarrely psychotic and self-destructive and required constant observation. When the parents applied for the patient's transfer to our service, which was nearer to home, we realized that we had nothing more to offer except a family approach, i.e., an approach that viewed the whole family as the real patient and the designated patient as only its symptom bearer or scapegoat.[2] Consequently, we agreed to accept the patient only if her parents were admitted also for at least a 2-week period.

A few hours after the joint admission, during which time the patient's homeostatic role in her parents' relationship difficulties had been discussed, she became virtually asymptomatic for the first time in many years, a condition she was able to maintain during the succeeding year, until her parents dropped out of outpatient family therapy. Both in the hospital and subsequently outside, the battle in therapy shifted from the patient's "sickness" to the powerful efforts made by her parents to avoid relating to each other in an emotionally direct manner.

With most of our family cases, the decision to admit the additional family members came about after a therapeutic stalemate had been reached. As with the cited example, the stalemate might have been reached after competent traditional treatment elsewhere had proved ineffective; in this kind of case we have urged family admission from the start. But in most cases (about 60 percent), additional family members were brought in after our own milieu approach had failed to promote significant changes in the initial patient's symptoms or social functioning. As we have become more experienced, however, we have increasingly requested family admissions at the time of the initial intake conference. Criteria for such a move will be discussed later.

In Bowen's early work in admitting the families of young schizophrenics, the parents spent their time taking care of the schizophrenic initial patient, but in the process they became overly dependent on the hospital and showed signs of regression.[3] To guard against this possibility and for positive reasons as well, our program charges each family member with taking care of himself, specifically with pinpointing and correcting his own relationship problems.

Starting with the initial intake conference and proceeding through the many subsequent therapeutic contacts, we repeatedly demand that the family member define his own problem, state his own goals for hospitalization, and outline the methods he will employ to achieve these goals. Even if he initially thought the purpose of his admission was to help his wife, son, or daughter with his or her problems, he is strongly urged to redefine his commitment to that of working on his own problems, with the understanding that any benefits that accrue to others are only happy by-products. Second only in importance to the fact of accepting admission itself, this redefinition is the key process by which the whole family and each individual member of it are made patients. The understanding is that each member has difficulties that contribute to the family disturbance but that each has the responsibility of differentiating himself from the sick family system.

The task of working on his own problems involves the family member in a many-hour-a-day job. Every day family members take part in at least one family therapy session, in which disturbed communication and relationship patterns are analyzed, and one individual psychotherapy session, in which current relationship difficulties are explored in terms of their possible reenactment of the individual's significant early relationships. In addition, there are ward meetings and group therapy sessions in which the family members are given feedback on their recent behavior by the whole therapeutic community and staffings and planning meetings in which the details of the individual treatment programs are continuously reviewed by other patients and by the staff.[4]

Role playing and psychodrama exercises are devoted to rehearsing more adaptive alternatives to the behavior manifested on the ward and in the group conferences. There may be specific behavior therapy exercises designed to remove old symptomatic behaviors or to develop new psychosocial skills. For example, certain fear responses may be modified through negative practice or systematic desensitization, and assertive behaviors may be successively approximated by modeling and operant cueing.[5] Programmed sensitivity exercises, such as the Human Development Institute (HDI) sequence for couples[6] and the Encountertape sequence for groups,[7] are presented as courses taken by most patients in basic communication skills.

Finally, every family member is held responsible for maintaining his room and for doing various ward jobs, such as arranging "buddy" systems for suicidal fellow patients, transporting food from the central kitchen, and planning recreational activities. He may also be urged to take a job elsewhere in the hospital if relevant social skill deficits can thereby be assessed and improved. All these treatment, educational, and work tasks are synthesized into a daily schedule cooperatively drawn up by patients and staff and modified as often as treatment progress dictates. Schedule breaking inevitably brings penalties, such as loss of privileges, extra work, and, if need be, discharge from the hospital.

During the period of the report when our overall average length of stay was 19.9 days, initial patients of families stayed an average of 16.8 days, and the additional family members 10.2 days. We have usually asked that family members stay only a week; frequently, however, they require several extra days to complete their tasks.

Case Reports

The following clinical vignettes illustrate the course of typical cases leading to family admission. Our most frequent situation is illustrated by the following report.

> *Case 2.* The initial patient was a 27-year-old housewife who had delivered her first child, a girl, 3 months previously. Although she was apprehensive about the baby she managed fairly well at first but then began to fear she would drop her child and prove inadequate in other ways. She withdrew socially, wept frequently, and just prior to admission began to fear that the neighbors were spying on her. In the hospital a regimen of phenothiazines and antidepressants was prescribed, and she rapidly improved. However, discussion of discharge led to a loss of initiative and a return of depressive symptoms.
>
> Although the patient's husband was noted to be quite schizoid about her difficulties at admission, she denied that he was anything other than a model husband. He was a graduate student in psychology, and he talked about her as a clinical case. It became obvious that he was her neutral therapist, she his all-compliant patient. Very indirectly she implied that after the baby arrived he devoted more time to his studies, leaving her when she needed him most. At the staff's insistence the husband entered the hospital; since the baby was well situated outside the hospital and the ward was full, her admission was not required.
>
> During the joint admission the patient worked on her nonassertiveness and her encouragement of her husband's emotional detachment by refusing to respond when he did show affect. This behavior was viewed as an attempt to recapture her early relationship with a depriving, aloof, and frequently hospitalized mother. The husband worked on abandoning the therapist role and showing more affective concern. Although a variety of treatment modalities were used, psychodrama with explicit modeling by the doubles seemed crucial in the treatment. The initial patient was able to accompany her husband home after 4 days, asymptomatic and committed to follow-up couple therapy. She has remained asymptomatic to the present and has required no special help with the baby. She discontinued outpatient therapy 2 months after discharge.

In the past we would have simply confronted this woman with her manipulative, regressive wish to stay in the hospital when her symptoms returned at discharge time. She might well have acquiesced and gone home to continue the covert battle with her husband, the outcome depending in large measure on whether she found competent outpatient help. The current approach gives more credit to the patient's communicative efforts and quite possibly curtails the length of aftercare.

The other most frequent type of family admission involves, as the initial patient, a borderline young postadolescent who decompensates after a first term away at college or after one or more serious failures in heterosexual relationships. The following vignette serves as an illustration.

Case 3. This 18-year-old attractive college sophomore entered the hospital after several mutilative suicide gestures (burning and slashing) following rejection by two successive boyfriends who disapproved of her manipulative sexual teasing. Her outpatient therapist referred her with the complaint that the patient responded to any penetrating interpretation of her behavior by threatening suicide. Immediately after admission she appeared perfectly poised and undepressed, but showed grossly inappropriate affect in describing her current condition. She was overheard accusing her mother by long-distance phone of "ruining my sex life." Yet she was resistant to having her parents come to the hospital and denied that she was any longer upset. In view of her real suicidal potential and inaccessibility to treatment, she was virtually forced to agree to her parents' flying out to Madison.

At the initial family conference it became apparent that the family was involved in a series of destructive triangles. The patient and her mother were, though both unaware of it, competing for the father's affection. In the process the mother conveyed great mistrust of her daughter's sexuality and constantly sought to undermine her self-confidence as a woman. In deference to her mother, the patient mutilated herself whenever her drives sought expression. The mother and father, on the other hand, had not been lovers for several years, and their relationship had degenerated into constant bickering from which the father usually walked away in a pout. The father and daughter were very obviously in collusion against the "bad mother," frequently giving each other nonverbal signs of support. It came out that the patient had gone on an eating binge and burned herself one year previously when her father had kissed her and complimented her appearance.

The family stayed in the hospital for 2 weeks while these various alliances were broken up. The mother and father self-consciously decided to turn to each other and to "throw their daughter out of the bedroom." When the patient tried to reinsinuate herself, the parents decided to leave the hospital and go back to their own lives with the aid of psychiatric follow-up. After a period of mourning, the patient accepted her new status and was able to return to school and begin dating boys on a more realistic basis.

This case illustrates well the resolution of the oedipal situation within a family therapy framework. With the environmental control afforded by the hospital, the loaded issues of who wants to do what to whom can be vigorously confronted, and then more realistic alliances can be formed and more realistic needs met.

Results

The authors rated all admissions on two main symptoms at admission and discharge. The symptom list included items such as disorganized thinking and behaving, suspicious or delusional thinking, excitement, and passive-agressive behavior.

We arbitrarily defined major improvement as at least a four-point reduction on a 10-point scale (0 to 9) in the primary symptom, to a final rating of 2 or less at discharge; moderate improvement was defined as a four-point reduction in either of the two main symptoms, regardless of the final rating. On the basis of these standards, 61 of the 100 index patients showed marked improvement; 25, moderate improvement; and 14, minimal to no improvement. During the same period 38 percent of the nonfamily patients showed marked improvement and 23 percent moderate improvement. These observations are preliminary to a statistically controlled study.

Discussion

Why family therapy in the hospital? Could not the family members have come for conferences on a once- or twice-a-week basis, as Gralnick and other hospital psychiatrists have recommended? [9] Are we not discussing a needlessly expensive and complicated procedure? This, of course, may turn out to be the case, and as yet we have no hard data to the contrary. But our enthusiasm is based on several considerations. First, we had reached an impasse with a significant number of patients whose key family members had been coming to the hospital once or twice a week but who abruptly began to make therapeutic strides once the family members were admitted.

As we have mentioned, the premise of family therapy is that the family and couple relationship system is primarily what is disturbed. The initial patient comes to medical attention because he is bearing the symptom or seeking help for the entire family. The reason he is selected may be due to a variety of factors: special sensitivities or vulnerabilities, birth order, appearance, genetics, and so forth. In actuality, the problem lies with all of the family, and progress in family therapy is predicated upon getting the various family members to accept this assessment. Thus both the suffering and the responsibility for change are diffused to a larger number of people who in aggregate are stronger than any one of them alone.

Our former method of involving families in a patient's therapy went contrary to this conception. It is clear that the casework method of seeing families mainly for informational purposes reinforces the split between who is sick and who is well, who is responsible and who is not. Sometimes the caseworker casts the parents in the role of villains, degrading the patient to the status of helpless victim rather than active contributor. No family therapy ever comes out of such an approach. The more sophisticated practice of having a hospitalized patient and his outpatient family members meeting together for conjoint therapy also undermines the family therapy premise, although much more subtly. They are all equally responsible; how can only one of them be treated without reaffirming the notion that he is really the sick one?

Having the family members enter the hospital, on the contrary, is a powerful act, realistically and symbolically. The spouse or parents thereby vigorously declare their status as fellow patients and coresponsibles. We are impressed with how often the initial patient's symptoms improve in the few hours after family admission. In about half our patients showing major symptomatic improvement, significant change occurred within 24 hours of the family's admission.

But just as important, the family group, once in the hospital, finds a degree of therapeutic intensity and control unavailable on an outpatient basis. Of the cases cited there would be little argument over the difficulty of managing the initial patients on an outpatient basis. In such cases the family patterns of relating are so ingrained and malignant that an hour or two of conferences per week is only piecework.

The most common criterion for the admission of "significant others" at the time of the initial intake is met when a marital partner's symptomatology impinges significantly on the life style of the spouse or threatens the perpetuation of the marriage, particularly when the presenting symptoms have been recurrent, long-standing, or unresponsive to individual outpatient therapy. Another frequent indication involves unmarried individuals whose emotional dependence on parents is so intense that they continue to rely on them for finances (this applies to most college students) or room and board into adulthood. Even if the patient's parents are divorced, we may still ask both to be admitted to the hospital. A special instance of parental dependence involves patients whose failure in love relationships or marriage can be construed as a reenactment of early maladaptive relationships to the parents. When a patient and his love partner are interviewed and their communications appear to be highly distorted by the presence of "ghosts in the room," we may ask that both sets of parents come for admission. In some circumstances of course we yield to practical necessity and settle for family conferences on a less intense basis than full inpatient status for all participants, but not when we feel that the intensity of the symbolism afforded by the act of admission is crucial to the therapeutic outcome.

Contrary to our expectations, we have found that family members show surprisingly little resistance to entering the hospital. Once the staff gets over its own ambivalence, the family members are usually more than willing, even at great personal sacrifice, to do something they can perceive as contributing to a definitive collaborative effort.

REFERENCES

1. Abroms, G. M., Fellner, C. H., and Whitaker, C. A.: The Family Enters the Hospital. Amer. J. Psychiat. 127:1363-1369, 1971.
2. Whitaker, C. A., and Olsen, E. H.: The Staff Team and the Family Square off. In: Abroms, G. M., and Greenfield, N. S. (Eds.), The New Hospital Psychiatry. New York, Academic Press, Inc., 1971.
3. Bowen, M.: Family Psychotherapy with Schizophrenia in the Hospital and in Private Practice. In: Böszörmenyi-Nagy, I., and Framo, J. L. (Eds.), Intensive Family Therapy. New York, Hoeber, Harper & Row, 1965, pp. 213-243.
4. Abroms, G. M.: Defining Milieu Therapy. Arch. Gen. Psychiat. 21:553-560, 1969.
5. Wolpe, J., and Lazarus, A. A.: Behavior Therapy Techniques. New York, Pergamon Press, 1966.
6. Human Development Institute: General Relationship Improvement Program, 5th ed. Atlanta, Human Development Institute, 1967.
7. Human Development Institute: Encountertapes. Atlanta, Human Development Institute, 1968.
8. Stampfl, T. G., and Levis, D. J.: Essentials of Implosive Therapy: A Learning-Theory-Based Psychodynamic Behavioral Therapy. J. Abnorm. Psychol. 72:496-503, 1967.
9. Gralnick, A.: The Psychiatric Hospital as a Therapeutic Instrument. New York, Brunner/Mazel, 1969.

PART V

GROUP TECHNIQUES

Developments in Transactional Analysis

by Stephen B. Karpman, M.D.

Transactional analysis is an ego therapy whose focus is clarifying relationships between people. It defines three basic attitudes of the ego: the Parent, Adult, and Child ego states. These three basic units may be presented graphically by a combination of circles and vectors so that transactions between people, however complex, can be illustrated with scientific simplicity. The vocabulary used in treatment is an outgrowth of the theory and must be understood by all three ego states. This must include the Child, and hence must be expressed with the concreteness, imagery, and fun that a child can understand.

For simplification here, the treatment will be presented as proceeding in four overlapping phases of increasing scope: structural analysis, transactional analysis, game analysis, and script analysis. Prospective patients are seen initially in several individual interviews and become familiar with the transactional approach through discussions and reading.[1-3] The treatment "contract" formed presents the cure point in a concrete and measurable way. The other patients in the group know what each patient's contract is and orient their questions toward this goal.

I. Structural Analysis

Structural analysis is concerned with the understanding and recognizing of ego states. All three ego states are normal and are always present or available, although only one is used at a time, just as only one TV channel can be used at a time. Ego states are objective social realities, not open to subjective interpretation, and diagnosable four ways: (1) body attitude, (2) tone of voice, (3) vocabulary, and (4) effect on others. Under special circumstances, an ego state can be contaminated, fixed, or decommissioned.[2] The three ego states are presented in their subdivisions below.

A. Dynamics: The Ego States

1. PARENT (P)

a. Prejudiced Parent. The prejudiced Parent stereotypes and labels people, thinks in terms of right and wrong and what people should or shouldn't do. The vocabulary includes words like "vile," "incompetent," "pesty," and "shameful." An erect stance with head tilted back and an accusing index finger are pathognomonic, as well as domineering, critical, pompous, or patronizing attitudes. This Parent has, on the positive side, pride, stoic strength, standards, and can present opinions.

b. Nurturing Parent. The body language shows a graceful flexion of the neck and a kindly, benevolent tilt of the head. The attitude is sympathetic, considerate, caring, concerned, forgiving, reassuring, understanding, and protecting. But too much, on the negative side, makes the person overprotective, "close-binding-intimate," oversolicitous, smothering, and infantilizing.

2. ADULT (A)

The *Adult* is the sensible, rational, logical, accurate, factual, objective, neutral, and straight-talking side of the personality. In computerlike fashion, problems are set up and solved, information is stored and memorized for later use, and best decisions are made from available information. The Adult keeps social control and decides which part of the personality to let out in varying situations. Too much Adult can be boring to the Parent and Child.

3. CHILD (C)

a. Free Child. This Child is happy, intuitive, spontaneous, natural, charming, adventurous, and creative. The fun and joy of the personality is here. Too much Free Child leaves the personality unprotected.

b. Adapted Child. The Child here is "adapted" in growing up to the mold of the parents' transactions. This ego state presents attitudes in the range of childhood feeling states, such as compliant, sulky, sad, spiteful, confused, sneaky, frightened, and guilty, in an exact replica of the original child reaction to the parents.

B. Treatment: Uses of Structural Analysis

a. To Learn the Ego States for Further Stages of Treatment. In initial individual interviews, the therapist uses structural analysis to clarify problem presentation. Illustrative questions are used, such as "What are your (Parent, Adult, Child) reasons for entering therapy? " and "How does your (Parent, Adult, Child) feel about this? " Some reading provides further depth, particularly Dr. Eric Berne's *Games People Play*[1] and Dr. Thomas Harris' *I'm OK.-You're O.K.*[3] In the first several weeks of group treatment the patient spends time practicing in spotting the ego states in himself and others in the group.

b. Know "Skull Transactions." There is a generally ignored internal dialogue between the ego states. In one conflict situation the Child may be saying, "I want to"; the Parent, "No"; and the Adult, "Let's work this out." In a depression, the Parent beats the Child repeatedly with, "There you go again." In defensiveness, the threatened Child says, "You take over," to the Parent, who then attacks the aggressor. A severely inhibited person who has "killed their kid" has to "run everything through their Parent" before acting. Transactional analysis (TA) gives permission to listen usefully to the voices in the head and gives "handles" and a sorting system for cataloguing this internal dialogue.

c. "Getting the Trash out of Your Head." This refers to the Adult decision to start a new internal dialogue to get rid of the bothersome "noise" of overthinking or the constant meddlesome effect of old Parent tapes. A "Go away" or "That's my Parent talking" often quickly helps a patient "divorce his Parent." A suicidal person finds he has a "kill yourself" playing over and over again on his Parent tape, and learns how to turn it off.

d. Reparenting. This refers to a regression stage in transactional analysis as applied in residential treatment of acute schizophrenics, where all old Parent tapes are erased and the mind is set free for a gradual reparenting with meaningful slogans and directives. Schiff [5] reports social cures in over 25 adolescent schizophrenics with the reparenting method.

e. Spelling Out the Sides to Your Personality. Most people have less than ten sides to their personality, and these can be very clearly outlined by the halfway point in treatment. This ego-state profile can be written on the blackboard, using an adjective or catchy slogan to describe the attitude, which is copied down for references by the patient. One housewife used four parental attitudes on her husband (for example, "You're only one millimeter long," "Schoolmarm," etc.), which she referred to as her "cutlery set." The group could refer to each one as it came up. Alcoholics universally use one of three Child "slip slogans" as they switch from Adult drinking to Child drinking. These are written on the blackboard as:

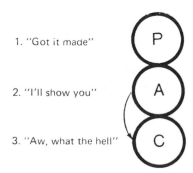

1. "Got it made"

2. "I'll show you"

3. "Aw, what the hell"

f. Setting Up Decisions. Choosing a mate can be aided by questioning to find what a person's Parent, Adult, and Child are looking for. One divorcee had a list of "non-negotiable demands" as follows: Her Parent needed a man who was (1) a social and business climber, (2) considerate and caring, and (3) aware. Her Adult wanted someone that could talk rationally; and her Child could only turn on to someone who was (1) tall and thin, (2) a "silly boy," and (3) a helpful Parent. Spelling this out cleared up for her why she always fell in love with the "wrong one" (her Child's choice) or always broke up with the "right one" (her Parent's choice). Another single woman, when asked what values in life were important to her, listed two Parent choices and one Adult one. This expanded into the "voting pattern" she used in deciding on men: two votes to her Parent, one to her Adult, and none to her Child. Another woman solved her long-standing inability to break up with a boyfriend. Her Free Child and Nurturing Parent liked him, her Prejudiced Parent and Adapted Child didn't, and her Adult was left indecisive with the 2—2 tie.

g. Who's Listening to Therapy. When treatment is not proceeding as rapidly as expected, it is discussed with the patient and he is asked to identify which ego state has been listening in therapy. If it was the Child, the patient may be getting confused or getting entertained by bright ideas (attending for a "treat instead of a treatment"). If it was the Parent, he may be getting information and rules with which to beat on the Child ("intellectualization") or gathering hostile stories about psychiatrists. The therapist, too, can check out which of his own ego states is listening in therapy.

h. How the Patients Sees the World. A patient's so-called illness may actually be the normal response reaction to his narrowed view of the world. It is quite effective in the early states of treating an inhibited person (playing "Wax Museum") to illustrate how few of his ego states are actually looking out at things, and how few of the ego states in others he is actually crediting them with.

i. The "Integrated Person." He has all the ego states available to him functionally. Treatment often pinpoints which side of the personality is not readily accessible and establishes a goal in therapy to reactivate those lost ego states. For example, the defenseless Child may need to bring out his Parent, the attacking tyrant Parent to switch on his Nurturing Parent, or the constant Adult to let out his happy Child. A poor conversationalist found out in therapy that she was withholding different ego states that had many interesting opinions, which she was not revealing to people. An artist's work didn't feel complete to him for the same reasons. One patient deliberately picked a job with supervisorial potential to develop his Parent in line with his treatment plan.

j. A General Sorting System. The P-A-C states can be used as a way of cataloguing external information. Movie critics can be judged on whether they watch with their Parent ("an important movie"), their Adult ("technical excellence"), or their Child ("uproariously funny"). Mental health books may be Parent (lists of do's and don'ts for a happy life), Adult (presenting information about behavior), or Child (entertaining without making points). Available psychotherapies can be catalogued similarly. Occupations have an appeal for the Parent (judge, nurse), Adult (science, accounting), and Child (arts, sports). Manufactured products and advertising are more acceptable if there is a positive appeal to all three ego states.

II. Transactional Analysis

TA deals with clarifying and diagramming the conversations between people. "Transaction" is used because "interaction" is considered a passive and vague word, whereas "transaction" illustrates the give-and-take specificity of exchanges. The stimulus-response verbal sequences can be diagrammed with arrows going from one of the ego states of a person to one of the ego states in another person, as in Figure 1. Ulterior transactions have transactions on both a social level and a psychological level simultaneously.

A. Rationale: The Transactions

1. SIMPLE TRANSACTIONS
a. Complementary Transactions. When the arrows between ego states are parallel, the conversation can proceed indefinitely. Examples: (1) Child→Child (fun talk); (2) Adult→Adult (straight talk); and (3) Parent→Child (helpful talk).

b. Crossed Transaction. The ego state addressed does not respond and there is a switch in ego states as well as a switch in subject discussed in the response. The arrows in Figure 1 appear crossed, as in the example from therapy below, where the stimulus is Adult→Adult but the response is Child→Parent.

2. ULTERIOR TRANSACTIONS
a. Angular Transaction. Three ego states are involved here; for example, a salesman's Adult is hooking the client's Child on the hidden psychological level, but is talking business to his Adult on the overt social level.

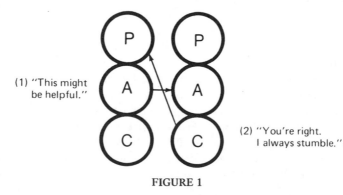

(1) "This might be helpful."

(2) "You're right. I always stumble."

FIGURE 1

b. Duplex Transaction. Four ego states are involved here; for example, an apparent Adult→Adult discussion on the social level "come see my etchings" on a date with some Child→Child fun being planned on the psychological level.

B. Treatment: Uses of Transactional Analysis

a. Communication Blocks. One couple could not solve their problems at home because they could not sustain an Adult→Adult conversation. His Parent thought her talk was "inconsequential" (Parent→Child) and his Child was frightened of her criticisms (Child→Parent). Meanwhile, her Child was trying to set up his Parent to be grandfatherly (Child→Parent) and her Parent was watching his ineffectualness (Parent→Child). It was always one of these four crossed transactions. When these were diagrammed the difficulty became clear.

b. How You Come On to People. This can be clearly illustrated by TA methods. Through group consensus, then blackboard illustrations, a patient's transactions in the group are drawn graphically, and can be learned by the patient as factual knowledge about himself. This will sometimes be the clearest he has ever "seen himself as others see him," and gives him a new awareness in his relationships.

c. What Your "Sweatshirt" Reads. A person's presenting identity can be summed up by the slogan emblazoned on the "sweatshirt" he or she wears in public, such as the Child "Nobody Knows the Trouble I've Seen" or the Parent "Don't Embarrass Us" A frigid woman wore the sweatshirt "I Wouldn't Want to Give Him the Satisfaction." Sometimes the back of the sweatshirt gives the slogan of what a person is like after you've known him awhile. One patient interviewed prospective boyfriends while wearing a sweatshirt with "Do You Qualify as a Husband?" on the front, and "Don't Leave Me," on the back. The slogan is easily recognized in therapy, either by intuitive summarizing or by latching onto a typical quote by the patient.

d. Typical Transactions. These can be learned just as typical games are. Usually they are Parent ›Child, and are illustrated on the blackboard. A slogan or a role name is written next to the ego state. Common ones are Bully→Clinging Vine, Bombastic Fool→Resistant Child, or one person with "mobility" and the other who is "stuck." These may or may not turn out to be role playing in a game or in a script, or to involve the therapist in "transference."

e. Options to Respond. Often people get into "locked" complementary transactions, and they can't figure a way out. Their options are one of many possible deliberately crossed transactions. For example, a person in a Child position says "I'm not" to a Parent repeatedly saying "You're bad." Some of the options are switch to a (1) Parent→Parent reply: "You're right. But it's the fault of the system. Let me tell you what the Telephone Company did"; (2) an Adult→Adult reply of "How so?" or "Define your terms"; (3) a Child→Child reply: "You're no bargain yourself" or "Go to hell"; (4) a Prejudiced Parent reply: "Stop that instantly!"; or (5) a Nurturing Parent offering, "Oh you poor thing. You've had a bad day. How's your asthma?"

f. Practicing Transactions in Group. From the work with the "options," a patient may find that certain ego states are not available to him and he will want to work on regaining their use. One "momma's boy" practiced being Parental in the group; a dictatorial Parent type practiced his Nurturing Parent, and a rigid Adult type was sent to "permission group" (a weekly play and encounter group) to "let his Child out." One patient could not hook other people's Adult into listening to him, so he practiced getting a "contract" to speak ("Get the floor") in the group before speaking.

g. Listening Blocks in Group. A patient who talks right through another person, or barely pauses to give a token imitation of listening and then continues with "As I was saying," can be interrupted, and the inaccessibility of his Adult can be graphically diagrammed. These "listening blocks" are all crossed transactions, and the importance of a person's realizing this is paramount for successful relationships. When the Child does this, it is often the helpless-Child-being-scolded ego state or the compliant docile Child who doesn't retain what's said. One patient who repeated herself endlessly thought the object of group was to "get through to people" and hadn't considered that people might want to get through to her Adult. Another patient was asked by the group to say "thank you for the useful information," to show that he listened to what was said. One angry Parent patient maintained he was pure Adult, despite the groups's seven to nothing vote that he was Parent, until he was asked to recall comments made to him, which his Adult couldn't.

h. "Transference." The question is asked whether transference comes up as a factor in an Adult-oriented, nonregressive group. It comes up occasionally and is handled as a crossed transaction. Sometimes it is specifically labeled as a "typical transaction" and the precedents are traced to early family transactions. When so labeled, it can be referred to again when it comes up later in group. Game and script transferences are handled similarly.

i. Seeing Others as They are. In discussing transactions one person may not be aware of the possibility of a reachable Nurturing Parent, Prejudiced Parent, Adult, Free Child, or Adapted Child in another. One patient, indignant about the "only" meaning of a remark made to her in group, was asked to review the possible positive intent by *each* ego state in the other person.

j. Understanding Transactions. In therapy, a patient sees that his problems do not exist in a vacuum. TA interpretations are bilateral, not unilateral, and include the outer world, (namely, another person) in each interpretation. One patient with a "Frankenstein" complex thought that his destructive, impulsive anger bubbling up from his volcanic id was his problem, but transactionally he had learned the scare games from his father, who worked with special police units. The bilaterality of relationships shows that if a person is boring you, it is because you gave them "permission" to bore you, or you are "bad" only if you are in the presence of someone who is calling you "bad." If you have an "unconscious," it is because transactionally you have to keep it unconscious.

k. The Relationship Diagram. This is used to show which channels of communication in a relationship are open and which are closed. A straight line is drawn between ego states in the transactional diagram to represent the nine possible channels of communication between people (that is, Parent–Parent, Parent–Adult, Parent–Child, etc.) A lasting relationship has at least half the channels open. A failing relationship may show loss of a previously open channel. For example, loss of a Parent–Parent channel (for example, widening political or religious differences), an Adult–Adult (can't discuss things anymore), or the Child–Child channel (less fun, less sex). The progress of a beginning relationship can be marked by adding each new channel that opens as people get to know each other better. The therapist-patient relationship can be drawn up to illustrate why some patients do well and some do poorly with a given therapist.

l. Pathological Transactions. Certain types of pathological transactions are emphasized when they show up in group. One is the "Gallows Transaction," in which the patient smiles and winks when he is talking of his failures ("Well, I think I took another step toward skid row last night, ha, ha.") and gets the other patients happily smiling back, thus acquiring group permission to continue on his failure script. Another is the "Discount Transaction," whereby Adult functioning is discounted by a Parent in the one of four ways:

a. There is no problem.
b. The problem is insignificant.
c. There is no solution to the problem.
d. Nothing can be done by me to solve the problem.

III. Game Analysis

Games are predictable, ongoing sets of transactions that proceed inevitably to a payoff unless interrupted. They are given names that instantly expose the Child: for example, "Now I Got You, You S.O.B." Each game has a characteristic number of players, and any player may play any of the hands in his game. Games can be played "easy" or "hard." Games are ulterior transactions with proceedings going on simultaneously at both a social level and a psychological level. There is a switch point in a game, after which happenings on the psychological level are felt in greater effect than the happenings that began on the social level. There are three game analysis diagrams and five principal payoffs of a game.

A. Rationale: The Game Diagrams

1. THE GAME FORMULA

$$C + G \rightarrow R \times S = P$$

or *Con* plus *Gimmick* gives the Response; then there's a Switch that gives the *Payoff*. The Con is the initial trick involved in the game. In the game of "I'm Only Trying to Help You" a person cons someone into helping him. The gimmick represents the other person's weakness that the con person has spotted; the Response is the help given; the Switch comes when the needy person kicks the helper, and his payoff is, for example, the look of justifiable indignation on the face of the helper. A sophisticated patient learns the "hooking" (irresistible urge) feeling of being drawn into a game; he knows the feeling of the Switch at the midpoint of the game, and the Payoff feeling after the game is over.

2. THE DRAMA TRIANGLE

"Karpman's Triangle"[4] (Figure 2) illustrates the sudden, dramatic role switches that go on in a game. Using the preceding example of "I'm Only Trying to Help You," the Victim (*V*) asks the Rescuer (*R*) for help. The Switch occurs when the Victim becomes the Persecutor (*P*) and the Rescuer is switched down to the Victim position. There are many interesting variations of this game in which the Rescuer winds up as the Victim. Another type of Switch occurs when the Rescuer switches over to the Persecutor position on the Victim. Another possibility occurs when the Victim winds up having to help his Rescuer, who claims to be a Victim. Drama can be light or heavy. An example of light drama is the father (*P*) who angrily sends the son (*V*) up to bed without dinner; later the son's dinner is brought secretly by his mother (*R*). In hard drama, a sexy patient seduces (*R*), her lonely psychiatrist (*V*), then switches to the Persecutor position, and reports this to all her subsequent psychiatrists, as well as to her friends, newspaper reporter, and lawyers.

Although the Drama Triangle is used primarily to indicate the Switches that

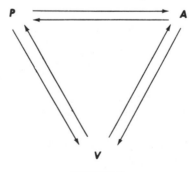

FIGURE 2

occur in a game, it also can illustrate the confusing possibilities of being hooked into the triangle so that once a person is in the triangle, he is switched rapidly among all roles, with the result that he is playing all roles at once. For example, a martyr mother sets herself up as a Victim of an unhappy life and nonappreciation by her children, sets herself up as the final Rescuer in the family by creating doubt as to whether the children can thrive competently on their own, and also as Persecutor, with constant pressure and guilt transactions.

3. THE TRANSACTIONAL DIAGRAM

The transactional diagram (Figure 3) illustrates with solid lines the apparent transactions visibly seen on the social level, and shows with dotted lines the more crucial transactions occuring on the psychological level. This illustration represents the "I'm Only Trying to Help You" game where there is an overt Adult→Adult request for help and the covert Child→Parent rejection of aid.

B. Rationale: The Game Payoffs

1. PROVE EXISTENTIAL POSITION

a. Childhood Decision. After a series of traumatic events in early childhood, the decision is made that, to preserve internal harmony, a position or stance toward the world must be taken to serve as a front line of defense. A game is played to continue proving that this decision is correct. Decisions are made, such as "I will have to go it alone without friends," which prevents risk of further letdowns, and the unhappy Payoff of the game is the proof of this position. The argumentative game of "Why Don't You—Yes, But" proves the childhood position of "Everybody wants to dominate me." In one case, a young girl, alternately treated lovingly on one day and beaten on the next by a drunken father, prevented future ups and downs by taking the position "All men are beasts," thus leaving her not vulnerable to men. The angry exchanges she would have with a male suitor following the rejecting game of "Rapo" proved again to her that all men are beasts. As with all decisions, these "decisions" can be reversed by therapy.

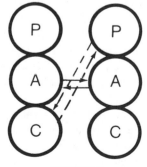

FIGURE 3

b. The OK Positions. People can take one of four basic positions toward the world, as listed below, The final result or Payoff at the end of a game proves one of these positions: For instance, a depressed person proves again that he is not OK in comparison to other people who are OK (item 3 below).

(1) I'm OK, you're OK.
(2) I'm OK, you're not OK.
(3) I'm not OK, you're OK.
(4) I'm not OK, you're not OK.

2. TRADING STAMP RACKETS

It was previously believed that people bottled up feelings until one day they would explode, but now it is thought that people save up different colored trading stamps and then cash them in for a desired prize at an intended redemption store. These are called Feelings Rackets, and games are played to collect the psychological trading stamps which are the currency of these rackets. For instance, a man needing only two more books of mad stamps comes home from work, starts a fight with his wife, collects the two books of mad stamps, and cashes them in at the bar for a justifiable drunk.

The four main colors for trading stamps are red stamps (mads), brown stamps (hurts), gray stamps (fear), and blue stamps (guilt). Most game players save up stamps only for small prizes; for example, 25 books of mad stamps are traded in the neighborhood bar for a week-end drunk, 25 books of hurt stamps are traded in at home for a week-end sulk, 25 books of fright stamps are cashed in at the neighborhood pharmacy for a free panic and tranquilizers, and 25 books of guilt stamps are traded in at the Emergency Room for a toy suicide attempt. People rarely save up for the biggest prizes (100 books): red stamps for a free homicide traded in at the morgue; brown stamps for a free quit of a job, marriage, or even the country, which can be traded in at the Canadian border; gray stamps for a free-go-crazy, which is traded in at the State Hospital; and blue stamps for a free kill-yourself, which is traded in at the coroner's office.

It should be noted that whereas most people feel bad for a while or handle their feeling at the moment, people in the Feelings Racket secretly save up all their stamps over a long period of time for a prize. In therapy, a patient learns to give up this trading stamp racket and to begin saving gold stamps (compliments). Twenty-five books of these are good for a free euphoria. One hundred books gives one permission to do something very big in his/her lifetime.

3. RECOGNITION STROKES

Strokes are the units of recognition and attention and are a biological requirement for survival. There are three main types of strokes: positive strokes, negative strokes, and crooked strokes. Many of these are given out at all times in games. A positive stroke is something done or said that feels good. Negative strokes don't feel good, but for people raised in families without positive strokes, games are played for negative strokes, as negative strokes are better than no strokes at all. Crooked strokes are negative strokes disguised as positive strokes. Patients raised on crooked strokes become suspicious of all strokes. Patients learn how to give up their negative stroke games in therapy and to give and receive positive strokes.

4. TIME STRUCTURING

There are only six possible ways a person can spend his time with other people; these are listed below in declining order of interest and stroking possibilities.

a. Intimacy. This is a very close moment of oneness with others when most of the channels of communication are open: for example, Parent trust, Adult frankness, and Child closeness.

b. Games. There is considerable interest and stroking in games, but the meaning and fullness of intimacy is lacking. People who are afraid of intimacy usually opt for games, and are reluctant to give them up.

c. Activities. There is a feeling of working together and a camaraderie during activities and work projects, but it is not so personal as intimacy and games.

d. Pastimes. Pastimes often include lively discussions of topics, issues, and current events, where most of the content has been prerehearsed or lifted from the newspapers for a topic of conversation. But it is fun and passes time. Pastimes in therapy, such as discussions of the weather, politics, or theories, seem quite superficial.

e. Rituals. People taking part in rituals are alongside each other, but are engaged in prerehearsed automatic behavior, with little creative opportunity or challenge or new personal confrontations.

f. Withdrawal. Withdrawal may happen with or without socially acceptable thought, when a game has been frustrated or given up suddenly before new Child activity has been discovered.

During the course of a day, people normally structure time in all the ways described above. In therapy it can be useful to analyze problem situations where there is an inordinate time allotment in any area. For instance, a married couple may spend all their time in activities, working on projects together, but have very few pastimes just for fun. Sexual time can be structured in any of the preceding ways: Sex can be intimate, or a game; it can be an activity for twice a week every week; it may be a pastime ("Ho hum, what shall we do tonight, dear"), a ritual ("Well, it's Saturday night again"), or withdrawal (impotence, frigidity, or none).

5. SCRIPT ADVANCEMENT

A person's Script is a preconscious life plan decided on in the Script Scene in early childhood. It takes a story form not unlike fairy tales, with a cast of characters and a dramatic sequence including Switch Points. Prohibitive parental injunctions narrow down a person's possibilities in life. Games push a person forward toward his script ending, such as the suicide ending in a lifetime "Kick Me" player.

C. Treatment: Uses of Game Analysis

a. Expand Psychological Awareness. The patient sharpens his thinking in therapy and becomes more aware of a wider range of richness in relationships, and meanings in his behavior. He sees that there are both social and psychological levels in behavior, that these two levels of behavior are possible simultaneously, and that possibly they have separate goals. He understands that there is surface behavior and behavior below the surface in others and in himself. He sees where a person's actions may relate to the past, to an unresolved childhood position; or they may be explainable by looking to the future, to the long-term goal he has set. He learns to delineate and circumscribe long chains of events and to label them comprehensively as a single entity. He learns that behavior can be oriented toward a Payoff and that games have internal psychological advantage, external psychological advantage, internal social advantage, and external social advantage.

b. Know "What's Going On." In contrast to some therapies that focus primarily inwardly on feelings, transactional analysis focuses primarily outward on the reality of "what really goes on" among people. The patient learns more and more about people through the TA books that are recommended and through the consistent focusing on the subtleties of the relationships between people in the group and of the outside relationships that they bring up to discuss. A certain psychological sophistication and perceptualness emerges. Some patients take a contract specifically in therapy to "find out what makes people tick" and see the reality of their relationships to others. A one-dimensional view of themselves and others is replaced by a three-dimensional view. The focus of a TA group is on people and what people do.

c. Know Feeling During a Game. The feeling of being "hooked" is described by some patients as an "irresistible urge," or a knowing that they are being "sucked into" something. One patient was angered by a reference to her in group as being "cheap"; immediately she went out and went to bed with a series of different men on successive nights. When she reported this in group the next week, a patient commented, "I'm surprised you got hooked so easily."

The feeling of surprise or devastation at a sudden Switch in a game can set an unaware person back for days. When patients report in group ongoing games that they are involved with, the group then discusses the possible switches in advance. This prepares the patient as well as gives him an overview of a game.

After a game is over, the patient is left with the Payoff feeling, to which he may succumb naively. He learns to see his part in initiating this so-called "unfortunate" happening and the repetitive nature of the situation in which he is left, and thus can face the decision of whether or not to keep playing games for that Payoff. One patient played several games, namely, "Blemish," "Kick Me," and "Debtor" all with the same Payoff of being left "lonely and out in the cold," in line with her "Little Match Girl" script.

d. Preventing Games. An aware patient, following his decision not to play a game again, can break up a game at several points or may decline to play. At the initial Con, when he is irresistibly hooked and drawn into the game, he may refuse to play or comment. Or he may anticipate the Switch in advance, discuss it with all concerned, and thus break off at that point; or he may realize that he has been hooked at the Payoff point and decide not to react further (that is, not use the Payoff to advance the negative aspects of his script). When a patient understands the game he plays, it becomes as easy for him not to become hooked as it is for other people who are not primarily game players.

e. Spotting Games in Therapy Groups. Games interfere with the straight transactions of therapy and are focused on when they come up. Games reported outside a group are commented on when they come up in group. Some patients use group therapy to collect trading stamps, which they then cash in for a free quit, a choice that advances their script by eliminating the hope of therapy. A patient is asked to "knock off the games" in therapy and get down to business.

Common games in therapy includes "Ain't It Awful" (but no mention of why the patient winds up in awful situations), "Psychiatry" (interesting intellectualizations and apparent progress, but no change), and "Why Don't You—Yes, But" (request for help, which is then rationalized away). Some games are exasperating to the group, such as "Do Me Something" (patient gives five words of partial information and then expects a complete answer in 50 words) and "Stupid" (group tries to pound the simplest idea into a patient's head). In individual therapy, a trained transactionals analyst can spot the different feelings the patient is hooking in him and inquire about a game this way. Ideally, the group with a wide variety of patient personalities provides the best setting for eliciting the range of behavior as it is seen on the outside in its natural form.

f. Eliminate "Most Destructive Game." A simplified short-term contract used frequently in group therapy and marathons is to help the patient find and get rid of his most destructive game. One young woman was suicidal and most destructive to herself in a predictable way following a game that was previously unknown to her. It began innocently with her asking for "advice," apparently in an Adult to Adult way. However, her Child hooked the helper's Parent, who then "took over" a Parent to Child relationship. The third step in the game occurred after a week or two of this in which the patient decommissioned her problem-solving Adult, felt futile, and sank into a morbid vegetative state, which fortunately the group could manage to bring her out of. When she was able to see that this series of moves in a game always preceded her suicide state, she was able to break up the game herself. Another patient, who often was beaten up and sometimes nearly killed through his hard game of "Kick Me," was able to delineate the three variations of the game he played; through social control he gained long-lasting, nondestructive relationships.

g. Building a Game. Sometimes in therapy the name of the game is not as readily apparent as the sequence of moves in the game. These moves are determined and listed on the blackboard and copied down by the patient for study. Sometimes a tentative name is given to the game. One patient found that her problems with dropping out of school, therapy, relationships with boyfriends, taking exams, quitting a job, and getting into debt, all occurred in the same predictable five steps. She could then interrupt these proceedings toward her Quit Point at any one of the five.

IV. Script Analysis

As mentioned previously, a script is a person's preconscious life plan decided on in childhood with the script decision. This decision, as with all decisions, can be reversed. Shortcuts have been devised in therapy to elicit the crucial script information, which is repeatedly clarified as therapy progresses until a patient can see a choice between keeping his old script and writing a new one. There are two main approaches used: The Script Matrix[6] charts the crucial parental injunctions that have served to narrow a person's possibilities in life. The other is the Script Story,[4] which gets a storybook picture of the patient's life pattern and predicts the ending to his script.

A. Rationale: The Script Matrix

1. COUNTERSCRIPT
This is an alternate script (Figure 4) and represents the "correct," socially oriented life goals the parents have indicated for the child. These injunctions come from the Parent ego state of both mother and father and tell the Parent ego state of the child what he should do. The first questions to a patient about what his parents wanted him to be usually produce counterscript information, such as "be a success," "go to college," or "live a happy life." People usually follow this counterscript, if they are shown how to do it, unless there are negative influences from the script.

2. SCRIPT
The true script message goes into a person's Child ego state, from the Child of the parent of the opposite sex. How to carry out this message is demonstrated

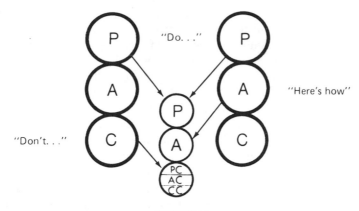

FIGURE 4

by the parent of the same sex ("Here's how" in Figure 4). The script Witch Message that comes in on the Child channel from the Crazy Kid in the parent is a negative, prohibitive injunction that becomes a limiting rule, which the Child ego state lives by. For instance, an injunction of "Don't Take Chances" would be triggered off in the patient's head whenever his Child is having fun, and would thus limit his self-expression and discovery. This is shown in Figure 4, using second-order structural analysis, with the arrow going into Parent of the Child (PC).

Sample "Don't" injunctions include: "Don't be in a hurry to grow up," "Don't do anything on your own," "Don't think," "Don't feel," "Don't be honest," etc. For a script cure in therapy, "permission" must be given to disobey these Witch Mother (or father) injunctions. The laugh of the "Gallows Transaction" is the Child laugh of the Witch Mother coming through. One patient laughs when she is sneaky in therapy, thus pleasing the "Don't be honest" idea of fun her mother taught her. One patient with a "Don't be happier than your parents" script stated that the turning point in therapy was permission "To be happy even though everyone around you isn't."

a. Fairy Tale. Patients are asked, "What was your favorite fairy tale when you were growing up?" and then asked to describe it as they remember it. This fairy tale will quite often reveal a pattern not unlike the patient's life pattern, and the parallels in the character roles, the traveling sequences, and the dramatic switches are easily seen. Sometimes his story is determined by tales of a favorite uncle, a favorite movie or book, or other story witnessed.

b. Tombstone. A patient can be asked, "What do you think will be written on your tombstone when you die?" He is asked to write on the front of the tombstone what he thinks should be on it, and on the back what other people would write. One patient was able to see his problem clearer after he realized that on the back others would write "Here lies a very well accomplished person," but on the front he would write "I wish life would have been completed." It turned out that this meant that he would have completed only what his Parent and Adult wanted to do, but his "Don't take chances" injunction was going to keep his Child from doing what it wanted to do.

c. *Script Sense.* The vivid, memorable event in early childhood in which a patient made a key decision that influenced the course of his life can be discovered in therapy. One older patient's depression was treated routinely by examining his relationships with people, until it was discovered that when he was young he made a decision that he would never again be back "on the other side of the tracks." Prior to entering therapy, he had to sell a piece of bankrupt investment property, but had underestimated the importance of this effect on him until he vividly recalled his childhood decision. One woman, whose problem was that she fought constantly with her husband, had made a childhood decision in an orphanage that "when I grow up, my children will not go without." However, the picture she had of being surrounded by the children did not include a husband. She admitted her husband's main complaint was that he always felt like an outsider.

d. *Build the Story.* Sometimes a person's life story has a recognizable story sequence to it, not unlike a fairy tale, with certain periods of inactivity (Sleeping Beauty, Rip Van Winkle) and travel to distant lands with a change in identity. Through familiarity with many fairy tales, the transactional analyst is able to assemble a story drama. One patient's phobias were traced back to a series of decisions he made as to how life would be different in the new "land" to which he was traveling, and this was similar to failure stories he had overheard as a child.

B. Treatment: Uses of Script Analysis

a. *Avert Tragic Ending.* Script analysis can predict the life course and dramatic ending of a script. One patient with a suicide script collected books of guilt stamps every week during group therapy. Discussion of her problems made her feel guiltier about them. Through discussion of her "No life after thirty" script and the collecting of stamps in group, she was able to use group for Adult purposes of getting well.

b. *Find Pervasive Life Influences.* Some patients who cannot give up a game, or who fight therapy without showing improvement, may be unknowingly influenced by a negative injunction or a script decision. One patient who decided in high school that henceforth he would hide his faults and fit in with all groups found that this script decision prevented him from revealing negative aspects of himself in the group. Others had not yet reached the point in their script where they were ready to switch back from a Frog to a Prince.

c. *Widen Scope of Therapy.* Script analysis provides a broader conceptualization than usually encountered in therapy. The widening of awareness to factors beyond the immediate problems expands Adult function. Alternate approaches to problems provide opportunities for breakthroughs in therapy.

d. *"Getting a New Show on the Road."* Transactional analysis aims to cure patients, not "make progress." Patients usually stay in therapy long enough to give up old unwanted script and "get a new show on the road." "Permission" in therapy is given to break the Witch Mother injunctions. This is followed by a necessary period of up to six weeks of Protection for the new ego, and this is dependent on the therapist having more Potency than the witch parents. Patients gain a final autonomy in therapy and choose their own style of life or even live "script free."

e. *Prevent "Hot-Potato" Scripting.* Through understanding of the script matrix and the influence of the negative scripting injunctions from the Witch Mother, patients gain new insight into the raising of their children. "Hot-potato" scripting occurs when a person passes his script on to his children or other people. One alcoholic patient with a "Don't think" injunction began explaining things to her six children, giving them permission to think logically as well as psychologically. The therapist should be alert to detect witch messages in his own script and should not pass these on to his patients.

f. *Life as a Fairy Tale.* The patient sees that he is living his life according to a childhood decision and not an Adult decision. Through therapeutic work with fairy tales, he sees the fairy-tale aspect of his life and recognizes how small a part reality plays in his decisions. Often it turns out that the therapist is a character in the fairy tale, and the patient's seeking of professional help was predetermined. With one Cinderella patient, the therapist was the "fairy godmother" through whom the patient would be transformed so that she would meet her Prince Charming and live happily ever after.

g. *Parental Wishes Outlined.* The script matrix provides a clear means of charting parental influences. Key messages are relegated to the three message slots in the script matrix. "Double-bind" and double messages are clear and separated, and show that the script message always takes final control over the counterscript message, all of which can sometimes be traced back through the parents to the grandparents.

V. The International Transactional Analysis Association

Transactional analysis was founded by the late Eric Berne in the 1950s. The ITAA was founded in the mid-1960s and is now composed of seminars and study groups in about 50 cities, with an active membership of over 1200 professionals. Meetings at the local seminars are held weekly or bimonthly. There are several grades of membership. A Clinical Membership is acquired after two years of supervised therapy and is approved by a board after a written and an oral exam. There is an annual summer conference, usually in San Francisco, California, in August. An annual Eric Berne Memorial Scientific Award is given for outstanding original work in Transactional Analysis. There was a quarterly *Transactional Analysis Bulletin* (1962–1970) and the *Transactional Analysis Journal* beginning January 1971. Transactional analysis became popularized by Dr. Berne's book, *Games People Play,* which was on the *New York Times* best-seller list for over two years. Clinical Members, with a Teaching Member standing, give lectures on TA and run workshops by invitation at various facilities around the country. Several cities have large training institutes and provide one- to two-month intensive training programs for learning transactional analysis group treatment. The mailing address of the ITAA is 3155 College Avenue, Berkeley, California 94705.

REFERENCES

1. Berne, E.: Games People Play. New York, Grove Press, Inc., 1964.
2. Berne, E.: Transactional Analysis in Psychotherapy. New York, Grove Press, Inc., 1961.
3. Harris, T.: I'm OK.-You're O.K. New York, Harper & Row, Publishers, 1967.
4. Karpman, S. B.: Script Drama Analysis. Trans. Anal. Bull. Vol. 7, No. 26 (April), 1968.
5. Schiff, J. L.: Reparenting Schizophrenics. Trans. Anal. Bull. Vol. 8, No. 31 (July), 1969.
6. Steiner, C.: Script and Counterscript. Trans. Anal. Bull. Vol. 5, No. 18 (April), 1966.

Marathon Group Therapy: Rationale and Techniques

by Ivan B. Gendzel, M.D.

The phrase marathon groups is frequently associated with concepts such as: transcendent experience, weekend orgy, nudity, affirmation, intimacy, precipitating psychoses, confrontation, attack, and genuineness. This presentation attempts to define what "marathon group therapy" does mean by initially comparing it to encounter groups and group therapy. The specific and unique advantages of this form of therapy are considered, and then a review of various techniques and the format of these groups is made. Finally, there is an overview of its worth in the therapeutic armamentarium, and the role of psychiatry in the marathon group movement.

Group Therapy, Encounter Groups, and Marathon Group Therapy

The use of group therapy as a therapeutic modality was initiated by Joseph Pratt about 1905 in association with his rest treatment of tuberculosis and has become an increasingly popular form of treatment, most particularly since World War II. A former consideration for the value of this experience was the ability to comprehend and experience a resolution of a transference neurosis. Factors which encouraged a movement away from this style of group therapy have included: an emphasis of ego psychology and a lessening of the relative importance of the classic and traditional analytic psychotherapies; an increasing existential and humanistic orientation; a general change in the conceptualization of mental illness with a tendency to deemphasize the medical disease model and with an increasing awareness of societal, family, and interpersonal relationships; the development of varieties of brief psychotherapies; and the desire of many for a more brief, inexpensive, and efficient form of therapy.

Under the aegis of educators and social and industrial psychologists, a separate small group movement started in 1946 during a short summer workshop and was encouraged by the subsequently formed National Training Laboratories. It emphasized the laboratory method of learning and research, and out of this movement new characteristics and philosophies of small groups have emerged.[1] These innovations and special attentions have included a here-and-now orientation, a marked emphasis on feelings and emotions, feedback procedures, interpersonal learning, and even formation of leaderless groups. Emerging from

151

this training group (or T group), and largely adapting its values and orientations, has been the encounter group movement. This has rapidly spread throughout the country so that every medium- and large-sized city, institutions of higher education, secondary schools, religious groups, and industrial organizations have had the opportunity to experience varieties of encounter groups.[2] These groups have also been called sensitivity training and human awareness, leadership training, Synanon games, psychodrama, Gestalt, nonverbal, and experiential. The particular emphasis on a style may vary, but the encounter group approach prevails. This current interest is attested to by the frequent appearance in movies, novels, newspapers, and magazines of material concerning these groups.

Time, one of the variables of any group meeting, has been adjusted so that some groups have been meeting for extended periods of time and have been labeled marathon groups. The sacrosanct 90-minute group therapy hour has been extended to include such time intervals as 6 hours, 12 hours, or more commonly 24 or more consecutive hours or several days with breaks for sleep. Early investigators have included Bach, Casriel, and Stoller,[3-11] who have helped to define the accelerated interaction said to be characteristic of this new format.

Rationale and Characteristics of Marathon Groups

Many of the general considerations concerning group therapy and encounter groups apply with equal validity to marathon groups. Confidentiality, physical restraints, no drugs or alcohol, and an attempt to present oneself honestly apply to most groups. What are the specific variables which, because of the extended-time feature, make for the unique contributions of a marathon group experience?

A marathon, unlike many open-ended groups, has two essential features:

1. A limited number of hours, usually more than 6, or perhaps 12 or 24 hours, a weekend, five 12-hour days, etc.
2. These hours are fairly consecutive and whatever momentum is built up is not allowed to dissipate during long periods when the group is apart.

The marathon group quickly becomes a world unto itself with a specific life-span. The participant is encouraged to accept the responsibility for himself and for his fate in the group. It is emphasized that there is some correlation between the paths he chooses in the group and those he chooses in the world. Importantly, he is made keenly aware that he has alternatives, and he is encouraged to risk attempting to find newer and perhaps better methods of relating with others. Change in the undesirable aspects of his presentation is acknowledged and approved by the group, thereby encouraging further attempts at change.

The time pressure helps to develop a sense of urgency and, coupled with a high motivation for being in such an extended group experience in the first place, a participant is usually willing to make an attempt to change. In addition to these considerations and to the frequent impacting of meaningful and demanding experiences, over the many hours a sense of fatigue builds up which further contributes to the dropping of defensive postures and facades. The sense of urgency, the high motivation, and the increasing fatigue are the specific factors which contribute to the uniqueness of the marathon experience.

Many other features have become associated with this experience. A more relaxed, informal setting, frequently a home, and the availability of creature comforts (such as food and bathroom facilities) make for a less artificial or clinical environment. Within this universe a group life emerges which is available to the scrutiny of all. Subgrouping, whispering, or experiencing meaningfully outside of the group is strongly discouraged. Within the microcosm that emerges, less and less attention is paid to the genetic antecedents; in contrast, the "here and now" is of greatest concern. Plans for the future outside the group might also be considered, but more important are plans for the future within the group. Frequently an attempt is made to draw up a contract as to what are the changes desired during the life of the group. A participant then has the benefit of experiencing directly his own changes and the effect of these on others. He is able to discover immediately the consequences of his actions, and to consider the desire of any further change.

A sense of belonging and cohesiveness develops during the course of the group. Attempts at "instant intimacy" do not succeed as well as allowing the group to experience for itself and to deal with its inherent stresses and strains and for members to accept each other and feel related. Intensive interpersonal confrontation and most particularly expressions of intense emotions accompanied by anger and tears appear to be part of the necessary steps toward achieving the desirable and necessary cohesiveness. Given the structure of the situation, the motivations of the participants, and the highly important role of the leader, this desired goal is generally achieved.[12-14]

The role of the leader is central to the group initially in setting the structure, defining the process, establishing the contract, and organizing for the event. Of equal importance is his role within the group as an active participant, an expert in interpersonal behavior, and a model for the others. Yalom states: "The curative factors in group therapy are primarily mediated not by the therapist, but by the other members who provide the acceptance and support, the hope, the experience of universality, the opportunities for altruistic behavior, and the interpersonal feedback, testing, and learning. It is the therapist's task to help the group develop into a cohesive unit with an atmosphere maximally conducive to the operation of these curative factors."[15]

Relative to ongoing weekly groups, the role of the marathon leader, as an involved participant and a model of expected behavior, is a more vital one, and more directly revealing of himself. The meeting may even take place at his house and with other family members attending. He shares his reactions and feelings with the group and, when appropriately stimulated, may feel free to express a problem area or a dilemma of his own. These have the tendency to make him all the more human and less the blank or aloof authority. As many studies in individual therapy have shown, it is this ability of the therapist to be involved and authentic, rather than autocratic and intolerant, which serves as a model for the other participants and encourages the honest and nondefensive behavior which helps to achieve the desired group goals. Each leader must develop an approach and a style of interaction that is unique to him. He should be a person with clinical experience, but without a "clinical approach." He should be a person acceptable to himself and with a desire to help others, and a willingness to be responsible, not only for his own behavior, but for the group and its results.[16]

Techniques, Methods, and Approaches

Specific techniques, methods, or approaches vary with the nature of the individual leaders.[3,10,13,17,18] No single correct methodology can emerge, and only a few techniques are enumerated here.

Instead of the standard question of "Why are you here?" a more precise definition and contract are required. Specifically, something of the nature "What is it you want to get out of this experience?" or "How do you hope to be different at the end of the group?" may be demanded of the participants early in the meeting. An answer is satisfactory only after it is acceptable to the rest of the group. Toward the end of the therapy the contracts are reviewed, and a final opportunity to fulfill the contract is afforded, or the contract may be modified.

Developments in electronic audiovisual media have allowed for the use of a variety of sophisticated instruments. Lighting effects and music as background to what is happening have been used effectively. For instance, flashing red and white lights with loud discordant music may accentuate angry words, and music as noise may be used to force a person to speak more loudly and forcibly. Sound and video recorders allow immediate playback,[19,20] unlike that from the rest of the group. Additional personnel, familiar with the equipment and the progress of the marathon, unobtrusively operate the equipment and are available as a resource for the leader or group.

Various encounter techniques, particularly as means of starting the group, are commonly used. These range from encouraging an individual to detail either the positive or negative impressions of some or all members of the group to encouraging participants in various risk-taking activities. Significantly, there is a marked tendency for nonverbal behavior to be observed, emphasized, and interpreted, and for varieties of this behavior to be encouraged. An example might be to encourage a participant physically to reach out for someone in addition to just making verbal contact with that person.

Varieties of nonverbal behavior might include the use of various art materials. The participants, either at the start or after a recess, might be asked to depict themselves by crayon or pastels on paper in any form or design in terms of how they then feel, and how they would like to feel at a later time. These drawings may then be individually presented to the group and discussed. Or two people may be asked to conduct a dialogue on paper without talking or writing any words, allowing one person to say something and the other person to respond until the conversation feels complete. At that point the two, either as a dyad or in front of the group, can discuss their "conversation" and how effective they were in communicating. Other materials, such as finger paint or clay, may be used for either individual activities, dyads, or larger groups.

The language of the body not only is listened to, but frequently is used as the major communicative form, particularly when the verbal mode becomes ineffective. For instance, two individuals who have reached an impasse and yet have not adequately resolved their situation might be asked to stand and face each other, to approach each other when ready, and then to have some variety of nonverbal interaction. The "variety" is not further specified. They are instructed to have this interaction until it feels complete and then to return to their initial place. These encounters might be very brief and involve only an exchange of an eye glance or handshake or may evolve into intense and prolonged interaction. The individuals then are asked if the encounter felt complete, particularly in terms of adequately communicating their feelings. If not, they are allowed to repeat it. The discussion that follows, both between the two participants and among the observers, lends further meaning and frequently clarifies how the verbal impasse had been reached. This interaction is particularly valuable between couples attending the meeting together. It may reveal and demonstrate to the others what could not satisfactorily be verbalized.

Another means of encouraging contact might be to ask people to stand and pair, then to face each other holding hands and closing eyes, and to try to become aware only of what the other pair of hands is "saying." The leader could then in a permissive manner encourage the hands to initially express anger, then to express warmth and affection, and perhaps even finally to explore the parts of the body to which these other hands are attached. Finally, the face could be explored and the partner helped literally "to open his eyes." The interactions would then be verbalized, initially with one another, and then with the group. This allows for an intense and significant physical contact between two participants, a chance to check the fantasied partner with the real one, and a chance to feed back to the partner the nature of the tactile impressions and how these correlate with the overall impressions of that person. A related activity might be "blind milling" when everyone, with eyes closed and arms somewhat extended, moves slowly about exploring his environment. This might serve as a prelude to the "hand conversation."

Schutz has compiled many of these exercises or situations.[21] As a means of attempting to free the person of his emotional impediments and of the physical expression by the body, Schutz carefully "listens" to what the body is "saying," encourages the bodily expression of feelings, and promotes the resolution of problems by a physical reenactment within the group. Examples might include learning to trust others by falling backward into their arms, or by having an isolated and withdrawn individual forcefully "break into" other social groups.

These and many other interactions become part of the group and may be used effectively if comfortably applied by the leader at the appropriate time. The rationale for these activities is that they provide an additional means to help set a more open and intimate tone within the group and also to circumvent the usual verbal barriers. Additionally, the satisfaction of being able to meaningfully communicate on paper or by hands serves a valuable function in terms of the group's interaction and the individual sense of accomplishment. Finally, information obtained can be conceptualized and verbalized and make a contribution to the overall marathon experience.

As the final hours of the marathon approach, the sense of urgency increases, the fatigue factor becomes more important, and the cohesiveness within the group is such that there is an even more meaningful and accelerated rate of interaction. There are various "go-arounds" with one person either telling the other individuals his reactions or receiving from all the other individuals their impressions. Almost always the participants, though physically fatigued, feel exhilarated and significantly related with one another as the group ends at its predetermined time. There is frequently a reluctance to separate, and any evaluations done at this time usually reflect the positive feelings and exhilaration of the person experiencing it. There are frequent comments about "let's keep in touch," and if a follow-up meeting several weeks later has been scheduled, reference is made to this.

The participants leave the marathon meeting in a certain "high" and with various expectations of change. The intensity of involvement and the degree of intimacy, however, are not generally available when the person "reenters" his usual situation, and a sense of disappointment is commonly experienced. This depressive episode or "down" usually comes on within several days after the marathon, and lasts for several days. If there is a follow-up meeting after several weeks, the participants will then frequently question the reality and worth of their initial experience and perhaps even comment about a dreamlike quality or unreal feeling or remembrance of the experience.

In summary the marathon group experience can be said to consist of three parts. Initially, there are the many events prior to the meeting, including any individual or small trial group experiences, and the obtaining of an informed consent by the participants.[22,23] Then there is the meeting itself. Finally, a follow-up meeting is usually scheduled. This is important in that it allows the participants to review somewhat more objectively and with the benefit of hindsight the intensive experience they have all been through and also allows provision for a sense of closure. Not uncommonly, relationships established during the meetings are continued subsequently, but the group as initially defined is terminated at this point.

Overview. Not every intense and emotional experience, even if it is labeled as a part of therapy, is necessarily corrective and desirable. Undoubtedly the structure of a marathon group does encourage and beget many intense emotional expressions, which hopefully benefits the participants, but this may not always be so. Attempts have been made to define what aspects of an encounter group experience are potentially most harmful, what individuals are most likely to be hurt by such an experience, and how to eliminate and "screen out" these potentially undesirable events.[22,24] Psychiatrists and inpatient units have had to care for people who have recently emerged from an intensive group experience and could not "put it all together." Here again, the ability of the leader is of paramount importance in initially screening out potential casualties, and also in evaluating and supporting such people once they are in the group. However, it has been shown that leaders are at times not as aware of the detrimental effects on a participant as are some of the other members.[24]

Whom should a psychiatrist refer for a marathon group experience? The patient might be someone "stuck" in individual or group therapy, or someone generally dissatisfied with his interaction with others or with strong neurotic tendencies which may benefit significantly from a marathon experience. However, a person with rigid or unyielding defenses or a strong need to remain isolated may be overwhelmed by these features and experience a detrimental disorganization. Though many factors enter into the selection, perhaps the most important are the motivation and informed consent of the person, and his awareness of his option to leave should he consider this desirable. (Though this is rarely exercised, the explicit awareness of this option may "permit" a person to remain and work through his anxieties.) Awareness of the opportunity to discuss this further after the group with a nonparticipant also helps to maintain a perspective on the experience and lessen the likelihood of an undesirable result.[24-26]

Are encounter groups to be considered group therapy, and is a psychiatrist in an encounter group a "therapist"? A task force of the American Psychiatric Association concluded: "In our opinion, a physician, even though he involves himself in a group nominally non-therapy in nature, still may not divorce himself from his traditional continuing responsibility to the participants whether or not they are specifically labeled his patients. [Members may join a human awareness group led by a psychiatrist because of covert expectations of a psychotherapy experience.] Encounter group trainers . . . are not legally responsible for possible detrimental effects of the group on a member unless the leaders are specifically advertised as mental health experts . . . it would seem probable that the psychiatrist retains his 'mental health expert' designation even when leading a group which is not specifically labeled as therapy, but which may be a potent influence, both positively and negatively, upon the mental health of the participants." [2][7] This implied burden of responsibility may partially help to account for the relatively lesser participation by psychiatrists in encounter and marathon group experiences.

But some other factors may be the specific medical model and training of a physician which appears antithetical to some of the desired traits of a group leader, e.g., clinical experience but not a clinical approach. The psychiatrist's traditional role is a distant, frequently enigmatic, self-reserving one, and more in line with the classically powerful, authoritarian, and sagacious physician. The trainer or leader is more self-disclosing and personally involved, with a willingness to be less of an authority. However, there are significant variation and overlapping in various leaders' and therapists' styles, and the specific professional background may be of less importance than the leader's clinical experience and his ethics and philosophy. In addition, since fatigue and inattention are likely, a cotherapist is desirable and a harmonious relationship between the two (or more) therapists is necessary.

What then may be expected after participation in a marathon group meeting? There is certainly no basis for a claim of an enduring and permanent change in one's personality pattern from this single event. Some have suggested that people periodically attend, perhaps at monthly intervals, a number of such meetings as a method of maximizing the benefits of the experience. Others have viewed the marathon meetings as a valuable adjunct to ongoing individual or group psychotherapy, as a diagnostic situation before therapy, or as an intensive means of getting involved in either individual or group therapy. Perhaps a realistic expectation of one marathon experience is that the participant would become more aware of his own feelings, experience a sense of well-being and relatedness to others, and acquire some insight which would make for more satisfactory functioning. For those in ongoing psychotherapy, the experience could provide valuable material to be further explored. Frequently important decisions are arrived at during the intensive meeting, and a proper balance between premature and impulsive action and, hopefully, a well-thought-out and advised plan of action are achieved.

This relates perhaps most specifically to marital problems made more overt during the meeting. If the pair is present, an opportunity is given for resolution; if one spouse is not present, a tendency exists to blame the spouse, particularly in view of the feeling of approval and acceptance the participant feels from the others at the meeting. Although divorce is an occasional outcome, there is more frequently a positive sense of commitment and affirmation to work constructively for fulfillment within the marriage. Most marathon participants benefit by having more of a positive sense of commitment in pursuit of their goals, particularly the interpersonal ones.

Marathon group therapy, then, offers a unique and powerful experience, the benefits and values of which are partially inherent in the structure of the group. The benefits also depend on the ability of the individual to assimilate the experiences both within the group and later, and on the skill of the therapist.

REFERENCES

1. Bradford, L. P., Gibb, J. R., and Benne, K. D.: T-Group Theory and Laboratory Method: Innovation in Re-Education. New York, John Wiley & Sons, 1964.
2. Rogers, C. R.: Carl Rogers on Encounter Groups. New York, Harper & Row, 1970, p. 9.
3. Bach, G. R.: The Marathon Group: Intensive Practice in Intimate Interaction. Psychol. Rep. 18:995-1002, 1966.
4. Bach, G. R.: Marathon Group Dynamics: I. Some Functions of the Professional Group Facilitator. Psychol. Rep. 20:995-999, 1967.
5. Bach, G. R.: Marathon Group Dynamics. II. Dimensions of Helpfulness: Therapeutic Aggression. Psychol. Rep. 20:1147-1158, 1967.
6. Bach, G. R.: Marathon Group Dynamics. III. Disjunctive Contacts. Psychol. Rep. 20:1163-1172, 1967.
7. Bach, G. R.: Group and Leader-Phobias in Marathon Groups. Voices 3:41-46, 1967.
8. Casriel, D. H., and Deitch, D.: The Marathon: Time Extended Group Therapy. In: Masserman, J. (Ed.), Therapies, Vol. 8. New York, Grune & Stratton, Inc., 1968.
9. Rachman, A. W.: Marathon Group Psychotherapy: Its Origins, Significance and Direction. J. Group Psychoanal. Process 2:57-74, 1969.
10. Stoller, F. H.: Marathon Group Therapy. Los Angeles, Youth Studies Center, University of Southern California, 1967.
11. Stoller, F. H.: Accelerated Interaction: A Time-Limited Approach Based on the Brief, Intensive Group. Int. J. Group Psychother. 18:220-235, 1968.
12. Dies, R. R., and Hess, A. K.: An Experimental Investigation of Cohesiveness in Marathon and Conventional Group Psychotherapy. J. Abnorm. Psychol. 77:258-262, 1971.
13. Gendzel, I. B.: Marathon Group Therapy and Nonverbal Methods. Amer. J. Psychiat. 127:286-290, 1970.
14. Sklar, A. D., Yalom, I. D., Zim, A., and Newell, G. L.: Time-Extended Group Therapy: A Controlled Study. Comparative Group Studies 1(4):373-386, 1970.
15. Yalom, I. D.: The Theory and Practice of Group Psychotherapy. New York, Basic Books, Inc., 1970, p. 83.
16. Rosenbaum, M.: The Responsibility of the Group Psycho-therapy Practitioner for a Therapeutic Rationale. J. Group Psychoanal. Process 2:5-17, 1969.
17. Ellis, A.: A Weekend of Rational Encounter. In: Burton, A. (Ed.), Encounter. San Francisco, Jassey-Bass Inc., 1970.
18. Mann, J.: Encounter: A Weekend with Intimate Strangers. New York, Grossman Publishers, 1970.

19. Berger, M. M., Sherman, B., Spalding, J., and Westlake, R.: The Use of Videotape with Psychotherapy Groups in a Community Mental Health Service Program. Int. J. Group Psychother. 18:504-515, 1968.
20. Damet, B. N.: Videotape Playback as a Therapeutic Device in Group Psychotherapy. Int. J. Group Psychother. 14: 433-440, 1969.
21. Schutz, W.: Joy: Expanding Human Awareness. New York, Grove Press, Inc., 1967.
22. Stone, W. N., and Tieger, M. E.: Screening for T-Groups: The Myth of Healthy Candidates. Amer. J. Psychiat. 127:1485-1429, 1971.
23. Gendzel, I. B.: Discussion of Stone and Tieger's Paper. Amer. J. Psychiat. 127:1489-1490, 1971.
24. Yalom, I. D., and Lieberman, M. A.: A Study of Encounter Group Casualties. Arch. Gen. Psychiat. (Chicago) 25:16-30, 1971.
25. A.M.A. Council on Mental Health: Sensitivity Training. J.A.M.A. 217:1853-1854, 1971.
26. Gottschalk, L. A., and Pattison, E. M.: Psychiatric Perspectives on T-Groups and the Laboratory Movement: An Overview. Amer. J. Psychiat. 126:91-107, 1969.
27. APA Task Force Report: Encounter Groups and Psychiatry. Washington, D.C., American Psychiatric Association, 1970, p. 22.

Large-Group Therapy with Multiple Therapists*

by Philip Herschelman, M.D., and David Freundlich, M.D.

Most group therapists concur that poetntial therapeutic success is greatest in small groups of approximately 8 to 10 patients, whereas, attempting to treat a large group of 35 to 45 patients is not only frustrating but of questionable therapeutic value. With the increasing popularity of ward or unit group therapy meetings, many a therapist has faced a large group of hospitalized patients and in the process has felt overwhelmed by massive patient resistance and hostility. More often than not he departs from this experience vowing, "Never again!" However, it is interesting to note how infrequently multiple therapists are utilized in such large groups. Many explanations can be given for this. For example, it could be assumed that too many doctors spoil the group. More precisely, diverse interpretations of group phenomena would result in confusion rather than clarification. Or the varying personalities, backgrounds, and needs of the multiple therapists would conflict and stimulate rivalry and staff dissention, rather than therapeutic cooperation.

In this paper the authors will describe their experience of working in a large group with multiple therapists. The emphasis will be on the reactions and interactions of the therapists in the large-group setting. It was our experience that the therapeutic success or failure of such a group hinges more on the feelings, attitudes, and interplay of the therapists than on the patients.

An attitude of skepticism permeated a group of psychiatrists working on the inpatient psychiatric service of the Philadelphia Naval Hospital when the unit head proposed that ward group therapy meetings be held which would be attended by the entire patient population and staff. The staff members remained pessimistic about the venture despite an agreement that only relatively limited goals would be pursued in the group, namely, reduction of ward tension by means of patient ventilation. It was hypothesized that a diminution of ward tension would make the patients' hospital stay more palatable as well as decrease acting out.

The group meetings were of 1 hour's duration and were held on the open and closed wards on a weekly basis. The sessions usually involved 35 to 45 patients,

---

*Opinions expressed herein are those of the authors and do not necessarily reflect the views of the Navy Department or of the Naval Service at large.

five staff psychiatrists, two or three psychiatric residents, two hospital corpsmen, and one psychiatric nurse. This was reducible to a ratio of one therapist to every 4 patients. Since it was impossible to seat everyone in a large circle, the chairs were arranged in loosely concentric ovals. The patient population was about evenly divided between the diagnostic categories of schizophrenia and personality disorders. The patient turnover was rapid with about 12 new patients arriving weekly. The usual length of hospitalization was from 4 to 12 weeks. Most of the patients were poorly motivated for therapy: their main interest was their future military disposition, that is, whether or not they would be discharged from the Navy or Marine Corps.

Early Group Meetings and the Aftergroup Group

In the initial group meetings there was considerable acting out on the part of the therapists. For example, whereas the patients were generally punctual, the therapists were frequently 5 to 10 minutes tardy. Another defensive ploy utilized by the therapists was passivity and nonparticipation in the meetings, this tactic being made easier because of the aggressive participation by the unit head. Although it was not clear initially, with time it became apparent that the therapists experienced intense anxiety directly related to participating in the group. Only with time did it become clear how anxiety-provoking and demanding the experience had been. As the therapists mastered some of their anxiety they gradually became more active and involved in the group. Initial resistance and skepticism gradually gave way to active participation and enthusiasm. Consequently, meetings spontaneously evolved which were held immediately following the large group sessions. On the open ward these were held in the presence of the patients, utilizing the staff-patient conference techniques proposed by Berne.[1]

The aftergroup groups were indispensable because they provided a forum where open communication between the therapists could be established. They proved especially helpful in resolving rivalry, anger, and various disagreements among the therapists. For example, one therapist irritated the others by his questioning of individual patients, much in the same manner as would be done in individual psychotherapy sessions. This technique frequently diverted the group from group affect and often resulted in a boring, intellectual dialogue between patient and therapist. When confronted about this technique in the aftergroup sessions, the therapist was able to reconsider his previously learned individual therapy techniques in favor of an approach which encouraged the expression of group affect and dealt with resistance in the group as a whole. All the therapists, to a greater or lesser degree, went through similar modifying experiences under the critical but supportive eyes of their colleagues. Although at times it was indeed painful to discover one's own flaws and weaknesses as a group therapist, nevertheless, an atmosphere of frankness and honest appraisal was maintained.

The aftergroup meetings were also helpful in exploring the change in attitudes of the therapists from initial resistance to active participation. All agreed that their initial resistance to participate in the meetings was merely a camouflage for their own fears. For example, most of the therapists openly acknowledged their concerns as to how they would appear as therapists in the eyes of their colleagues. The aftergroup groups, therefore, were an important learning experience for the therapists in that group therapy technique, counter-transference, and therapist interaction could be discussed.

The Technique, Advantages, and Problems of Multiple Therapists

In the large group meetings it soon became evident that an even dispersal of therapists about the room contributed to a secure feeling among both the patients and staff and made it easier to deal with destructive forces in the meeting. The need for this became glaringly apparent when it was observed that some patients frequently arrived early in order to manipulate the seating. For example, there were meetings in which patients diagnosed as character disorders sat together in one section of the room. As the meeting progressed this seating arrangement proved to be extremely disruptive. Despite the presence of many therapists, this cluster of resistive patients became impenetrable and resulted in decreased group interaction. This problem was solved quite simply by one or two therapists merely approaching such a group at the beginning of the meeting and requesting that particular patients exchange seats with them. When the therapists were evenly dispersed throughout the group, each was able to keep an eye on the small group of patients seated in his immediate vicinity. The acting out of a character disorder or the bizarre behavior and verbalizations of a psychotic patient could thus be handled by having those patients sit next to a staff member. For example, if a patient attempted to carry on a private conversation with his neighbor, a therapist in that vicinity would invite those patients to share their thoughts with the entire group. Sometimes when the meetings became charged with feeling, those patients who were not participating found it difficult to continue in silence. No longer able to vent to their neighbor, they often became active participants in the meeting.

Another lesson learned early in the large-group experience was that the therapists were much more effective if they behaved as "real" people who expressed their own feelings. Many of the therapists were apprehensive about assuming this role since they had been accustomed to being more detached observers during psychotherapy sessions. This type of withholding approach in the large-group meetings usually resulted in similar behavior by the patients. On the other hand, when the staff more freely shared feelings and reactions with the patients, the latter felt more confident about doing the same. This atmosphere was also conducive to helping the patients become aware of how they came across to others. In addition, patient identification with the therapists was enhanced when the therapists allowed themselves to be real "living" persons in the group meetings. Therapist-therapist interactions, therapist-patient exchanges, and the variety of therapeutic personalities present resulted in an expanded base available for patient identification. At the same time the functioning of the therapists as real persons was of benefit in destroying the patients' myth (and frequently the staffs') that the therapists were omnipotent and omniscient beings.

One of the striking advantages of multiple therapists was the enhanced ability to confront and quickly deal with patient resistance so as to readily reach significant, affect-laden material. In the group meetings the patients were simply not allowed to dwell on resistive topics such as hospital regulations, society, and the world political scene. In an assertive fashion the therapists redirected the discussion to the here and now of the ward setting and the group. For example, one therapist might say, "Okay, that's the situation in Vietnam, but what's happening in this room?" Or, if appropriate to the particular meeting, another therapist might interject, "Are we at war in this room?" Despite the use of an aggressive therapeutic approach, instances of patients losing control or of extreme impulsive behavior were unusual. Even on those occasions when anxiety became intense and a patient would begin to leave the room (on the pretext of having to go to the toilet), it was usually possible for the therapists to persuade him to remain in the room in order to discuss his resistance to the group situation.

With multiple therapists present, it was quite natural for one of them to follow up and reinforce a meaningful interpretation made by a colleague that would otherwise be lost in a sea of resistance. For example, when a particular group meeting would become intellectual and vapid, therapist A might comment to the group, "I'm feeling bored—what's happening?" Some patients, fending against significantly underlying affect, might collectively disagree that the meeting is dull. At this point other therapists, who were experiencing the same boredom, might reinforce therapist A's interpretation of the tone of the meeting. Frequently, this resulted in subsequent patient corroboration and exploration of the resistance. More often than not there followed an unfolding of intense affect that had been disguised by the aforementioned resistance. In a similar situation a lone therapist would probably find it extremely difficult, if not impossible, to meet and break through such strong resistance.

Another asset of multiple therapists was that different therapists manifested varying sensitivity to the wide spectrum of group phenomena. Therapist B, for example, would pick up a significant covert group affect that therapist A had missed altogether. Or therapist C would point out group interaction at a more superficial level, whereas therapist D would detect group affect at a deeper level. When such situations arose and as the therapists themselves became more comfortable with each other, it became possible for one therapist to lead another away from less productive to more productive areas. On occasion it was deemed appropriate for one therapist to disagree flatly with another. In such a situation it was not at all infrequent for the therapists to become angry with one another; however, with open communication being encouraged by all, the angry feelings were invariably resolved either during the large group meetings or in the aftergroup sessions.

Although all the therapists were considered to be of equal stature in the meetings, some therapists invariably felt more comfortable, and thereby functioned more therapeutically, in certain group situations. Some were more capable of handling anger or depression or of uncovering resistances. Other therapists were more adept at being supportive and reassuring to patients when the group situation indicated that approach.

> A vivid example of how a particular therapist handled a situation in more therapeutic fashion than his colleagues is illustrated as follows. In one group meeting, just before the Christmas holidays, the predominant feeling was that of gloom and despair. A heavy, steamy atmosphere permeated the room. It was all too easy to sink down in one's chair and say nothing. The meeting went slowly with little said and many silences. No one focused on the predominant affect of despair. Finally, after approximately 40 minutes, one patient became extremely angry and blurted out at the therapists, "You're no doctors!" He accused the staff of making extra money for each additional patient that could be kept in the hospital over the holidays. Most of the therapists responded angrily and met his attack with verbal counterattacks. However, one therapist was able to sidestep the accusations and point out that the patient was upset because he and the other closed-ward patients would not be spending the holidays at home with their families. The therapist added that one way of handling despair and depression in such a situation was to become angry, especially with those held responsible for their retention in the hospital. The patient in turn nodded agreement and ventilated his despair about being confined in the hospital. Other patients then did the same and there resulted a significant dissipation of group tension and partial resolution of the despair.

In addition to the many advantages of the multiple-therapist technique, numerous problems also became evident. On occasion the therapists, especially when anxious, talked too much, thereby inhibiting spontaneous interaction by the patients. When frustrated in their therapeutic attempts, the staff sometimes banded together "against" the patients, consequently reinforcing patients' resistance. At times, some therapists dominated their colleagues, and, conversely, some therapists found it all too comfortable to be passive and to relinquish active participation to others. The physicians were generally more active than the attendants, the latter often feeling insecure, inferior, inadequately trained, and, therefore, less capable of therapeutic contributions. Frequently, the staff prematurely assumed the full responsibility of setting limits on acting out behavior during the meetings, instead of sharing this responsibility with the patients. Since the patients were living together on the ward it would have been more important for them to learn how to confront and deal with each other's disruptive behavior, rather than unnecessarily depending on the staff to do this. It should be mentioned that most of these countertransference and intertherapist problems were transitory and were usually successfully resolved in either the large or aftergroup meetings.

Discussion and Results

The impact of the large-group therapy meetings with multiple therapists exceeded the initial expectations. There was appreciable evidence that the meetings resulted in greater benefits than simply reducing ward tension and patient acting out and making the ward a more pleasant temporary home. The group, as a whole, learned that certain emotionally laden areas could be explored without courting disaster. Some of the topics that were first defended against but later uncovered and discussed in the group were: loss of self-esteem from being a mental patient in a "nut house"; feelings of helplessness and hopelessness usually related to the patients' confinement to the closed ward; fear of becoming "crazy" or living with others who "act crazy"; anxiety concerning death, self-destructive impulses, and suicidal attempts; and apprehension about losing control of impulses. For example, the patients with character disorders frequently were hostile toward and avoided the most psychotic patients. There was evidence that the character disorder patients fantasied that too close contact with psychotic patients would result in uncovering their own imagined psychoses. When this phenomenon was acknowledged and dealt with in the group, there was a noticeable breakdown of barriers between the character disorders and psychotic patients. The psychotic patients in turn, as would be expected, were especially sensitive to and upset by group phenomena related to loss of control. It was frequently observed that when a particular impulsive patient was confronted in the group, several psychotic patients invariably disrupted the meeting with fragmented verbiage. Through the collaboration of the multiple therapists the focus would be redirected to the threatening area, which would then be discussed. One area generally avoided by the group but clearly part of some meetings was anxiety related to homosexuality.

Although it was impossible to determine to what extent intrapsychic changes occurred, it was obvious that many patients developed a better understanding as to how they came across to and affected others. For example, patients who often complained of being "picked on" and "harassed" began to see how their own provocative behavior often stimulated retaliatory responses. Thus, a good number of patients were able to modify their behavior and thereby elicit more friendly and receptive attitudes from others.

Of course, not all patients were helped in the group meetings. Certain hard-core character disorders strongly resisted all attempts to get them involved in the group. Another patient type that undoubtedly derived minimal benefit was the extremely withdrawn psychotic patient who rejected all invitation to interact in the meetings.

The large-group meetings not only were therapeutic for many patients, but also proved to be most helpful to the therapists in their work on the ward. Despite transient jealousy and hostility encountered among the therapists, the predominant attitude and feeling throughout the multiple-therapist experience was that of the cohesiveness, group identity, and a spirit of working together. The increased communication among the multiple therapists during the group and aftergroup meetings led to a striking improvement in staff morale. Furthermore, during the meetings the entire therapeutic team was able to sense the ward atmosphere, to become acquainted with the patients assigned to the various therapists, and to develop sensitivity to potential ward problems.

The utilization of multiple therapists in large-group therapy meetings was found to be a significant improvement over the traditional ward meeting or patient-staff conference. The initially limited goals of reducing ward tension and acting out by means of patient ventilation were surpassed. Despite the size of the meetings it was often possible to explore significant affect-laden areas. The aftergroup meetings contributed appreciably to the therapists' professional growth and to the general morale of the therapeutic team. The multiple-therapist technique could provide an additional and effective treatment modality in many institutional settings characterized by a large patient-therapist ratio, and where treatment is usually restricted to chemotherapy and ward milieu.

REFERENCES

1. Berne, E.: Staff-Patient Staff Conference. Amer. J. Psychiat. 125:3, 42 (September) 1968.

A Follow-Up of Ur Adaptations in Private Hospital Patients

by Monte J. Meldman, M.D., Rudolph G. Novick, M.D.,
Morris B. Squire, B.A., and M. V. Ostrowski, M.A.

After broad-based individual and group therapy at a private psychiatric hospital, 326 questionnaires were sent by mail to 187 female patients in the 18-65 age group who had been treated for a minimum period of 2 weeks during 1964 and to 139 who had been treated during 1969 for a wide range of behavior disorders. The questionnaires, modified from the Sheppard and Pratt Hospital forms, were designed to elicit data as to current physical or mental symptoms, interpersonal relationships, job performance, and social interaction.[1] Only 37 members of the 1964 group responded, whereas 99 members of the 1969 group did so. In order to obtain further information from more patients, the remaining members of the 1969 group were contacted by telephone, and an additional 20 replies were obtained, constituting 119 total replies in the 1969 group, an 85 percent return. The returned questionnaires were classified as to the current status of the patients as "good" result, "fair," or "poor" according to the following criteria.

The "good" group consisted of patients who were no longer in psychiatric treatment, were symptom free, were functioning at a healthy level with no emotional or physical complaints, and had shown improved work, family, social, and interpersonal adjustment.

The "fair" group included patients who were still in treatment and taking medication, but who experienced less morbidity from their symptomatology, and still had difficulties in work, social, and interpersonal functioning.

The "poor" group consisted of patients who were still in treatment, were taking medication, had the same or increased symptoms for which they were hospitalized, and evidenced decreased performance in work and in group activities with more withdrawal and impaired functioning in social and interpersonal relationships.

All of our "good" patients had received individual psychotherapy, 76 percent community group therapy, 40 percent somatic therapy, 10 percent EST, and 94 percent specific chemotherapy, of whom 89 percent received tranquilizers and 50 percent antidepressants. On follow-up, only 12 percent of these patients were still taking such medication whereas 72 percent of the "poor" patients remained on medication after discharge. Average duration of hospitalization was 1.7

months for patients who improved and 3.8 months for those patients who did not.

Findings

Of the 119 patients who responded to the questionnaire, 47 were classified as having achieved "good" improvement, 42 "fair," and 25 "poor."

The latter group was characterized by recurrent physical symptoms or had actual organic disease which had not responded to psychiatric hospitalization.

Of the 47 members in the "good" responder group, 12, or 25 percent, specifically mentioned a reawakening of faith and religious experience, as did 8, or 21 percent, of the "fair" responders. None of the poor responders mentioned a recurrence of religious awakening in their therapeutic progress. Our studies showed minimal correlation between original diagnosis and degree of recovery.

Discussion

The results of this preliminary investigation into the effectiveness of hospital treatment provide data that are consistent with the development of all three Ur adaptations (renewed physical, social, and psychologic confidence[2]) as an important factor in recovery from mental illness. Trust in their physician as a healing source was mentioned by approximately one-half of the patients, and those who were cured of their illness expressed renewed social optimism; 20 responders also had a more intimate relationship with their deities that they attributed to their hospitalization. The following are typical responses.

"My stay at the Forest Hospital has taught me a great deal in handling my small problems which all of us must have today to cope in our troubled times. I have a dear and understanding husband, wonderful friends and neighbors, and, best of all, family. I have found my identity as a person and human being. I thank God every day that I am alive and well."

"Although I am behind in my work and each week brings added duties, I am happy for I try to tell others about my God and how He can deliver them from all their tears and troubles."

"Maybe my footnotes may not help others, but I do know and firmly believe that positive thinking and faith in God's will is and was my best medicine."

Summary

The data from an investigation of the results of hospital therapy were examined for the efficacy of Ur adaptations as reported by patients in a questionnaire study and were particularly noteworthy in patients who achieved a maximum degree of improvement. The Ur defense of religious faith was the most frequently encountered factor in the reports from patients who achieved complete remission of symptoms, increased work efficiency, and improved familial and social adaptations.

REFERENCES

1. Whitmarsh, G. A., and Schutz, C. G.:A Follow-up Survey of Admissions 1960-1964, The Sheppard and Enoch Pratt Hospital. Res. Rep. No. 5 (November) 1969.
2. Masserman, Jules H.:A Psychiatric Odyssey. New York, Science House, 1971.

PART VI

COMMUNITY PSYCHIATRY

Therapeutic Abortion Trends in the United States

by Abraham Heller, M.D.

The modern era of medical abortion practice in the United States started only a little over five years ago when the state of Colorado led the nation in updating its 100-year-old abortion law.[1] The history of the passage of the act through the Colorado legislature is a saga worth retelling.[2] The attack was spearheaded by a brilliant, young, first-term representative. The bill was reported out for consideration by the legislature under a list of sponsors who already comprised a majority of the members of both legislative chambers. All major arguments against the proposed legislation were anticipated, and counterarguments were effectively marshaled against them, both in the legislative debate and in the public media. The bill passed relatively intact by comfortable majorities, and the governor signed the new law.

The debate had been at times highly emotional and even acrimonious. Deeply entrenched values and traditions, with religious overtones, were involved. All states and the District of Columbia had these century-old laws, which derived mainly from two sources. One was the Judeo-Christian cultural value system, which has traditionally sanctified human life and procreativity. In addition the old laws were devised actually to protect women; the surgical arts required for abortion a century ago were crude and dangerous.

Individual doctors had lent invaluable support in the legislative debate in Colorado, but organized medicine put in no presence. Following the passage of the law, medicine found itself quite unprepared and exhibited caution and marked indecisiveness. Organized medicine was clearly sensitive and defensive. Dire predictions had been made putting organized medicine on notice lest Colorado become the "abortion mecca" for the nation when an amendment limiting abortions to state residents was beaten down in the legislature. Thereupon the state medical society adopted a provision in its guidelines which discouraged abortion service to out-of-state residents. Many practitioners and hospitals were leary of the charge of "abortionist," which had the impact of an epithet. For many other practitioners a complicated personal and professional adjustment needed to be made, and this would take time.

The new law itself proved to be not really as liberal as supposed. It was patterned after the model of the American Law Institute. Abortion practice still remained part of the criminal code. Abortions could be performed only in accredited hospitals, only for reasons of threat to life or grounds of serious and permanent impairment of physical or mental health. Also, the law allowed abortion on humanitarian grounds in certain cases of rape and incest. For psychiatric indications, a psychiatrist had to certify as to "serious, permanent impairment." Then a special board of three other licensed physicians, not necessarily psychiatrists, was required independently and unanimously to approve. The law was undoubtedly the best that could have been passed at the time, but it set up complicated mechanisms to ensure the retained interest of society that no woman should receive an abortion except for the most serious reasons. This difficult system has proved time-consuming, costly, and discouraging to many women.

Nevertheless, with all the professional conservatism and indecisiveness the consequences of this still-bad law have been sweeping and momentous. Far more important than the local clinical impact has been the influence of the Colorado experience on the country as a whole. Discussion of abortion issues has built up to a sustained volume in both the professional and lay press across the country. Hardly a day passes but what the news media contain columns and reports on the subject. We have stopped keeping track of the rapidly lengthening list of medical, paramedical, legal, and religious, and other organizations which have taken formal stands in favor of liberalized abortion laws. Now 15 states have passed new abortion laws. Most have continued to pass laws based on the model of the American Law Institute, as did Colorado, but three states have legislated in effect abortion upon demand—no longer "therapeutic abortion" but legalized "medical abortion." Unquestionably many more states will follow suit with some new law in short order. Also, Great Britain and Canada have enacted new progressive legislation. These English-speaking countries and the United States exert mutual influence on each other. And finally the problem is being attacked frontally in the courts. Cases are in process in many sections of the United States which may very well overturn all the remaining old laws and many of the new ones on the grounds that it is a free right of the woman and a free right of her physician to decide together as an act of private medical practice whether she should have an abortion.

Denver General Hospital Experience

At DGH until May, 1967, about one therapeutic abortion a year had been done. At the present time the rate seems to be approaching 500 per year. In passing from virtually nothing to 500, the road has been hard. There have been many more problems than meet the eye.

From May, 1967, through July, 1970, a period of 38 months, the DGH Therapeutic Abortion Board evaluated 699 cases and approved abortion for 457 and disapproved 242. Until relatively recent months the approval/disapproval rate ran roughly 60 percent/40 percent. Now disapproval has dropped significantly to about 20 percent. The Board has manifestly become more "liberal" with experience and more accepting of broader grounds for approving abortion. A few of the disapprovals were not recommended by the referring psychiatrists; a few more were based on legal technicalities; but most represented a difference of opinion between the board and the psychiatrist as to the proper judgment in applying the law. Occasionally the board in disapproving sympathized with the needs of the woman, even the viewpoint of the psychiatrist, but felt he had not adequately documented his case.

Roughly 70 percent of this series of therapeutic abortion applicants had family income below $6000 per year or were on welfare (Figure 1). Forty percent of the applicants belonged to ethnic minorities, black or Spanish background (Figure 2). The data tell two things at once. Whereas in America traditionally the public hospital, virtually the only resource of the poor, has given little or no therapeutic abortion service, the situation at DGH is significantly changed. Considerable numbers of the poor are for the first time availing themselves of therapeutic abortion. But poorer women are characteristically slower to be aware of and to take advantage of health opportunities. Conversely, middle- and especially upper-class women always could bend local resources to their advantage, or go elsewhere. Denver General has been aspiring, at the same time, to a broader image as a community hospital giving high-grade service to all regardless of ability to pay, not discriminating any more against those who can pay than against those who cannot. Hence women of means, who might not use Denver General for other medical needs, have turned to DGH as a hospital where therapeutic abortion applicants would be evaluated "liberally" compared to the rest of the community.

One straitforward conclusion, by those of our persuasion, would seem to be that family health counseling, family planning with therapeutic abortion as one available strategy, should be stepped up among the poor and ethnic minorities. But unfortunately there are complications which are reflected in the stand most recently taken by the National Medical Association in which black physicians are primarily represented. On the one hand, therapeutic abortion, the association holds, should be a private matter between the woman and her physician. But the association goes on to warn that we must guard against therapeutic abortion turning into a means of genocide. One philosophy holds that the breaking of the poverty cycle depends on such vital factors as raising health standards, that the "healthy mother—healthy child" sequence and interaction (a concept being

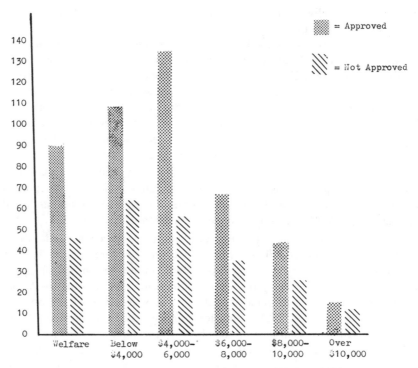

FIG. 1. Economic class, Denver General Hospital, May, 1967-July, 1970.

Family Income	Approved	Not Approved
Welfare	90	48
Below $4000	109	61
$4000-$6000	133	57
$6000-$8000	67	37
$8000-$10,000	42	27
Over $10,000	16	12
TOTAL	457	242

strongly promoted by the American Medical Association) is indispensable to this process, and that the healthy mother—healthy child complex can be significantly enhanced by the availability of therapeutic abortion. Some ethnic minority leaders, however, take angry exception and assert that so-called therapeutic abortion is a ruse by means of which the establishment majority intends to decimate the ranks of the minority poor. Thus, deplorably, the matter is politicized. In our direct experience, however, minority women are just as anxious as any and all others for free and easy access to therapeutic abortion (TAB).

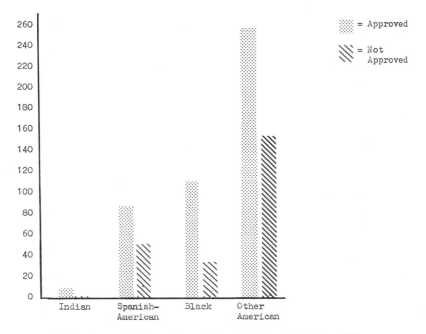

FIG. 2. Ethnic background, Denver General Hospital, May, 1967-July, 1970.

	Approved	Not Approved
Indian	5	0
Spanish-American	84	50
Black	108	34
Other American	260	158
TOTAL	457	242

Contrary to earlier studies which showed utilization of TAB predominantly by married women, in our series over half the cases were unmarried teenagers, and a majority of them were not emancipated from their families (Figure 3). The married woman with intact family, and therefore with more life supports, experienced a higher rejection rate from the board.

In contrast, there has been a growing tendency in our hospital as in the rest of the state, as well as in the other states with new practices, to view unwanted pregnancy in an unemancipated teen-ager as strong, *ipso facto* evidence of "serious, permanent impairment" of mental health. The theory is that during these critical years, in this state of immaturity, the impact has profound and far-reaching effects, frequently victimizing the girl who was unequal to the pressures which got her into difficulty in the first place. The counterargument is usually that to maximize the potential for responsibility in the girl the board

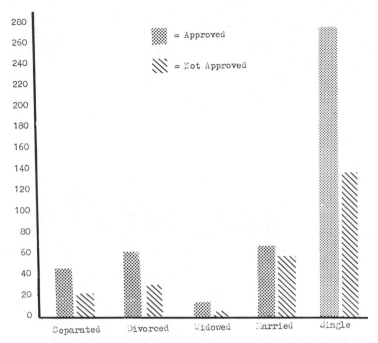

FIG. 3 Marital status, Denver General Hospital, May, 1967-July, 1970.

	Approved	*Not Approved*
Separated	45	20
Divorced	60	28
Widowed	12	3
Married	62	59
Single	278	132
TOTAL	457	242

ought to help her face and not remove the consequences of her behavior. In the favorable tendencies of board members in these cases one can see elements of chivalry (board members are virtually universally men), elements of parental projection (what parent is not uneasy these days about his teen-age daughter?), as well as elements of mental health objectivity (Figure 4).

About two-thirds of the series gave "Protestant" as religious affiliation. About 30 percent more were Catholic. (See Figure 5.) These ratios reflected fairly the religious distribution in the general population of our region. The evaluating psychiatrists have been very sensitive, seemingly more sensitive than the patients themselves, lest Catholic religious background contribute to the neurotic potential and adverse sequelae in consequence of abortion. Our Catholic patients have most often taken the position that they considered that

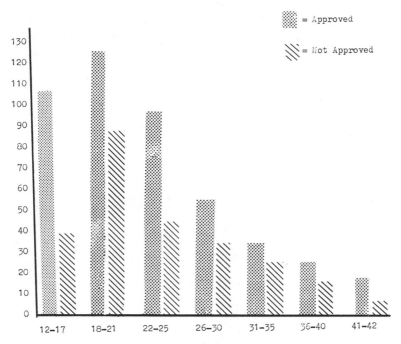

FIG. 4. Age, Denver General Hospital, May, 1967-July, 1970.

	Approved	Not Approved
12-17	108	39
18-21	127	89
22-25	97	43
26-30	55	31
31-35	31	23
36-40	23	13
41-42	16	4
TOTAL	457	242

there was little or no conflict for them between their religious convictions, such as they were, and what they felt were overriding reasons for wanting and needing abortion. In most cases denial was not notably present in these patients. Neither in the immediate postabortion period nor in follow-up to date have we noted any untoward experiences on this score.

Over 90 percent of therapeutic abortions done at DGH have been for psychiatric indications. Diagnosis of major psychiatric illness has been exceptional, hardly more than 1 in 10 cases. A greater number have had some psychiatric treatment in the past. Fewer were in psychiatric treatment when

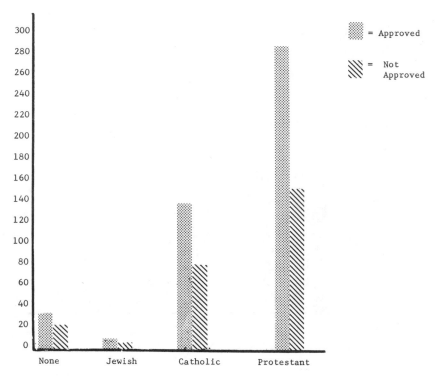

FIG. 5. Religion, Denver General Hospital, May, 1967-July, 1970.

	Approved	Not Approved
None	32	19
Jewish	5	4
Catholic	138	75
Protestant	282	144
TOTAL	457	242

unwanted pregnancy supervened. A fair number had had manifest psychological difficulty, for example attempted suicide, at some time in their life, untreated more often than treated. But fully half or more had no history of previous psychiatric disorder or treatment.

No consensus or guidelines existed as to what might constitute "serious, permanent impairment" of the mental health of the woman whose pregnancy is either wanted or unwanted. Some practitioners preferred to have convention set by medical or psychiatric societies. But this was resisted by those who preferred to allow convention to distill in time in the free course of practice left to judgments of individual practitioners and boards.

Some psychiatrists wished to confine the psychiatric qualifications under the law to cases of major illness only, others to conventional diagnoses of mental illness of serious degree. But many felt that conventional diagnoses were inadequate to subsume the broader mental health issues at stake. This kind of viewpoint has been eloquently expressed in "The Right to Abortion: A Psychiatric View," by the Group for Advancement of Psychiatry[4]:

> Motherhood is a task that requires enormous human and emotional resources. It is an obligation that confronts and challenges the woman's capacity to care night and day. Done in the spirit of love and fulfillment, it is hard but rewarding work. But when the child is unwanted, the task may become onerous and obligations created by such motherhood may become a lifetime sentence, an ordeal emotionally destructive to the mother and disastrous for the child.

At DGH, TAB patients are hospitalized on the maternity floor. What was once 1 TAB to 1425 births in a year, now is approaching possibly 500 TABs per 2300 births. Juxtaposition of aborting life and bringing life into the world among other incongruities in accommodating a new practice on an old service resulted in difficulties for both patients and staff. Special inservice training for staff and extra consultation by a psychiatrist and a psychiatric nurse were required to bring the problem to adjustment.

Less than one-third of the DGH therapeutic abortions were done prior to 12 weeks of gestational age. (See Figure 6.) This group was usually done by the dilatation and curettage method. Only recently has the suction technique been introduced. The remaining three-fourths of the cases were usually done by hypertonic amniocentesis. In these cases the risk of morbidity rises notably. There have, however, been no deaths from therapeutic abortion to date in our hospital, and none reported also for the rest of the state.

The psychological course of the therapeutic abortion experience is a function mainly of the state of the patient plus the age of gestation. The more intact the patient, the better she tolerates the procedure. The sicker the patient, the more morbid is her psychological reaction to the abortion procedure itself. A schizophrenic woman, for example, may become transiently more floridly psychotic. Also, the more advanced the pregnancy, the more physically stressful is the operative procedure. Not alone is there physical stress, but there have been bodily and psychological changes as well in the patient giving the pregnancy, the unborn, more "reality." Hence the psychological stress increases. Sensitive, supportive, psychologically skilled management, even treatment, may be very helpful. Adjunctive psychotropic medication is very helpful, especially in florid psychotic states. Even our sickest patients regain equilibrium in a matter of days. The most usual reaction is a brief, transient, mild, occasionally moderate depression. We have had no known major adverse sequelae to date.

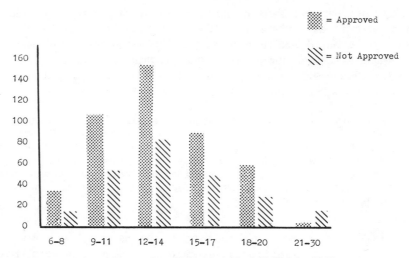

FIG. 6.   Gestational age, Denver General Hospital, May, 1967-July, 1970.

Weeks	Approved	Not Approved
6-8	35	15
9-11	113	53
12-14	158	81
15-17	87	48
18-20	60	27
21-30	4	18
TOTAL	457	242

Before we embarked on our clinical experience of now more than three years we were made anxious by our reading of the then classic literature which overemphasized the traumatogenic potential of therapeutic abortion. Our experience is in total agreement with the latest position of the American Psychoanalytic Association, joining so many other professional associations in urging removal of medical abortion from the criminal statutes averring the relative psychological safety of the abortion procedure.

Colorado Statewide Experience

The first consequence of the new law in Colorado was inhibitory rather than facilitatory. Although the grounds were presumably liberalized, the process was made more "responsible," that is, in fact more formal, more complex, and more difficult. Yet the best estimates are that TAB increased eightfold in the first year.[3] But this increase was mainly confined to Denver, the metropolitan center of Colorado, alone. Of the state's more than 50 accredited hospitals, less than half appointed or activated a therapeutic abortion board, and only three or four really got involved in the practice.

In 1967 when the new law was first passed, three hospitals did 90 percent of the reported therapeutic abortions in the state. In 1968 five hospitals did 85 percent. In 1969 the same five did 80 percent, and in the first 6 months of 1970, 75 percent. It follows, therefore, that other hospitals are becoming more active. The list of hospitals with any involvement at all is slowly growing. Other hospitals are shifting in TAB activity from low to intermediate gear.

In the first 12 months after the passage of the new law (May, 1967, through April, 1968) it is figured that over 400 TABs respectively were reported to the state health department, as required by another new law which had by then gone into effect sharpening the legal obligation to report TABs. However, our feeling is that TABs are not being fully reported, and therefore these figures are low. The first 6 months of 1970 alone already show 842 TABs. The projection for annual 1970 rate, at the same rate as the first half, would be 1684. (See Table 1.) So, considering the estimate of 50 TABs a year prior to the new law, we could compute an increase in annual rate of TABs of 3368 percent, or roughly a 34-fold increase. So perhaps progress is being made.

The population of Colorado rose 25 percent during the last decade, or perhaps 2.5 percent a year. Total births, on the other hand, had been declining through 1967. Then in 1968 and 1969 births rose again, about 15 percent and 5 percent respectively. Then in the first half of 1970 births showed a reverse again, down 5 percent. (See Figure 7.)

The ratio of therapeutic abortions to births for the first year was about 1 percent. In 1969 it was about 2.5 percent, and in the first half of 1970, about 4.5 percent. (See Table 2.) These ratios are still nowhere near those obtained in Japan and Eastern Europe. But the rate in Colorado is rising markedly. The 1970 total will unquestionably approach 2000 cases. If the legal attack which is currently proceeding in a Colorado court succeeds, abortion on demand will become available, and the medical abortion rate will rise even more sharply.

Over the state as a whole it is clearly perceived that both medical practitioners and hospitals are becoming more accustomed to therapeutic abortion practice and increasingly taking a more relaxed attitude toward it. The judgments as to what clinical conditions qualify under the law are clearly

Table 1

Colorado Health Department:
Reported Therapeutic Abortions

Table 2

TABs/Births, %

Colorado Health Department: Reported Therapeutic Abortions		TABs/Births, %		
1968	497	(12 months)	5/67-4/68	1.1%
1969	990	(12 months)	1969	2.5%
(projected) 1970	1684	(6 months)	1/70-6/70	4.5%

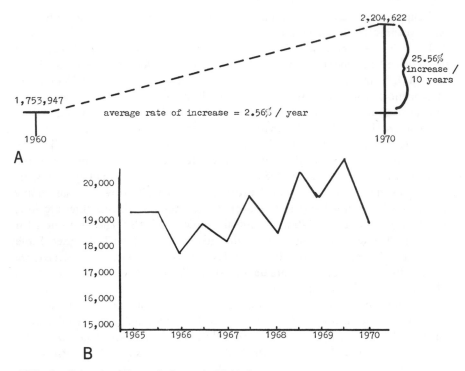

FIG. 7.   Colorado (A) population and (B) births.

Colorado Births

	Jan.-June	July-Dec.	Year Total
1965	19,165	19,172	38,337
1966	17,569	18,661	36,230
1967	17,980	19,327	37,307
1968	17,968	20,405	38,373
1969	19,248	20,912	40,160
1970	18,389		

becoming broader and more flexible. Again, it is the group of single teen-age girls who receive the greatest benefit from this liberalization judgment.

Over the state in 1968 80.2 percent of the cases reported listed psychiatric grounds. In 1969 73.4 percent gave psychiatric grounds, and for the first half of 1970, 86.7 percent were psychiatric.

Difficulty was experienced in other hospitals as well, as it was in DGH, over any significant number of abortions being handled on a maternity service. The two practices do not mix well, and putting them together causes trauma and divisiveness, for patients and staff, among themselves, and between each other. It has finally come to appreciation that any significant increase in therapeutic abortion practice will put a strain on services not geared for it.

Nationwide Implications

Abortion is still an emotion-laden issue. But reform and change are inevitable. It is only a matter of how quickly and in what form. Some states will continue to pass reform laws, such as may broaden the allowable grounds for legal abortion, but leave the restrictions in the criminal code. This kind of reform is already considered anachronistic. Some states may pass reforms which transfer the question of legal abortion, still retaining restrictions, sometimes relatively narrow restrictions, to the medical practices code. Such acts are philosophically more acceptable, but are practically little different from the criminal code laws.

Some states will retain the independent review board. This mechanism may be effective in safeguarding the interests of society, where it has any. But boards' functioning are full of vagaries and inconsistencies. Moreover, the interests of the patient whose case is presented *in absentia* are not well represented in board considerations. The board system delays, complicates, and otherwise inhibits the abortion process.

Then some states will repeal current restrictive laws and leave abortion open to restrictions only of standards of medical practice. Or the courts may strike down restrictions and leave medical abortion as a right of the woman to procure or a practitioner to perform abortion in meeting the rights and needs of his patients.

Legal reform will not by itself really solve the problem of constructive abortion services for women. Clearing away the legal restrictions merely uncovers a new set of problems. The medical profession is conservatively conditioned against broader abortion practices. Doctors and paramedical professionals have an enormous problem in adjusting to the new demands. The medical delivery system is already overburdened with ongoing services. The transfer of any significant number of women into legal, medical channels for abortion will create a number of pressures, not the least of which is inflationary.

The question is always raised as to whether extension of medical abortion cuts down nonmedical or illegal abortion. There are no hard data as to how extensive illegal abortion practice is. The best estimates are that nonmedical abortions run 25 percent of births. If millions of women are to be transferred from the illegal, nonmedical channels to the legal, medical services, this will cause a crisis which is already being experienced in some areas, notably New York, for the total medical establishment.

Organized medicine has the responsibility to prepare for the inevitable flood of therapeutic abortion traffic. Such preparation will undoubtedly require new and specialized services. If the woman can be channeled to a decision swiftly and directed into the medical system early in the pregnancy career, then therapeutic abortions can be done safely and economically on an outpatient basis. Such services are currently rare in the United States.

Population control has only recently become a concern in the forefront of the minds of the American people. So far it can be said that medical abortion has had little impact on population in this country. Is the reversal of the birth rate in Colorado, downward if only for a brief period despite a manifestly increasing population, meaningful? The time period is too short to tell. But the number of abortions in Colorado is beginning to be significant. The downtrend, if it is sustained, will undoubtedly be due to a number of influences, but probably therapeutic abortion plays a real part.

The Colorado State Health Department statistics indicate that about two-thirds of the reported therapeutic abortions in the state are "illegitimate." We presume this means not only pregnancies in single girls, but also pregnancies in divorced and widowed women. But the never-married young girl is the one who comprises the vast majority of this whole group. There can be little question that the increase in therapeutic abortion practice in Colorado is making a significant inroad in the number of so-called illegitimate births. The same could be expected for the rest of the nation.

The Women's Liberation Movement in the United States has seized upon abortion on demand as one of its demands. Clearly masculinist attitudes or outright misogyny has been imprinted onto the life of the United States, as in most countries and cultures, since probably the beginning of time. Availability of therapeutic abortion contributes importantly to the social, economic, psychological, and possibly physical freedom of women.

The changes in the medical abortion area are happening very rapidly. The role of the psychiatrist should be to lend the support of scientific, professional, and other objectivity to the process of changing the attitudes of societies and its subserving institutions, as well as individuals, to upgrade the quality of life, again, for individuals and society as a whole.

REFERENCES

1. Colorado Revised Statutes, 1963 (1967 Suppl.), 40-2-50, 51, 52, 53.
2. Lamm, R. D., Downing, S., and Heller, A.: The Legislative Process in Changing Abortion Laws, The Colorado Experience. Amer. J. Orthopsychiat. 39:684-690, 1969.
3. Droegemueller, W., Taylor, E. S., and Drose, V. E.: The First Year of Experience in Colorado With the New Abortion Law. Amer. J. Obstet. Gynec. 1035:694-702, 1969.
4. The Right to Abortion: A Psychiatric View. Group Advance. Psychiat. VII(75):203-204, 1969.

Techniques of Social Systems Intervention

by Paul Polak, M.D.

A social systems approach implies that a neurotic symptom may transmit a pointed "state of the union" message about a core family conflict at the same time as it expresses an individual's internal conflict. Each level of social organization, from the individual through his family and his neighborhood, functions as a subsystem of a larger organization, and conflict may be expressed at various organizational levels. Psychiatric syndromes represent one form of communication about social systems conflict.[1-7]

The crisis intervention service at the Fort Logan Mental Health Center treated over 1600 psychiatric patients by intervening directly in social systems disturbances in the patients' real world settings. The 2 to 25 people who are routinely involved in assessment and intervention procedures include family members, neighbors, employers, or friends, representing disturbances in the home, neighborhood, school, or work.

Concepts of Social Organization

A social system consists of two or more individuals who interact. This definition includes highly structured, relatively persistent systems such as social agencies or schools, as well as informal, transient systems such as a group of teen-agers watching a street fight. It includes the small system of the childless married couple and the larger system of the neighborhood in which the couple live.

The concepts of therapeutic community described by Maxwell Jones and others[8,9] are applicable to a wide variety of social systems outside psychiatric hospitals. Learning theory concepts fit naturally into this framework. The following specific areas form a useful basis for conceptualizing social processes.

Leadership. Many systems disturbances, from family crises to upheavals in the administration of large public institutions, can be traced to conflicts in leadership and power. Effective intervention in such disturbances must be based on a rapid appraisal of the formal power structure of the organization, present patterns of leadership and leadership conflict, and the evolution of leadership within the system. Leadership patterns often evolve through repeated upheavals in the distribution of power and the roles of leaders in the system. Unless *all* the individuals in formal positions of power or informal positions of influence in a social system are directly involved in the process of change, constructive change is unlikely to occur.

Role. Role conflicts are common determinants of social system disturbances.

> One family was seen after the teen-age son shot and killed his father in a hunting accident. After the death, the mother expected her son to be the host for social gatherings with her friends, whereas he expected her to be both a sports companion and a firm disciplinarian. Grief work with individual family members had to be integrated with a family process of clarification of the role that had been filled by the father and reassessment of those aspects of his role that could realistically be assumed by the survivors.

Communication. The patterns of communication within a social organization form the substrate for internal and external transactions of the system. Our practice is to call together all members of a system in a face-to-face meeting and ask them to talk to each other about a subject significant to the system. The customary verbal and nonverbal communication styles are readily observable and usually predictive of the structure and function of the total organization.

The degree of discrepancy between overt and covert communication with a system is often a reliable predictor of disturbances within the system. High discrepancy is often associated with the occurrence of psychiatric illness and antisocial behavior on the part of systems members.

Reinforcement Patterns. Each social system tends consistently to reward some patterns of behavior of its members and punish other behavior. This is especially pertinent to psychiatric illness. Many observers[10,11] have described a variety of transitory psychiatric symptoms as concomitants of life crises. Our observations suggest that such psychiatric symptoms persist and become identified as psychiatric illness when they occur within a rewarding social matrix. The act of hospitalization may remove a patient from an illness-reinforcing matrix, but unless the reinforcement patterns within the patient's real life setting are altered, he runs a high risk of recurrence of psychiatric symptoms at the first crisis following his return home.

Social Systems Assessment

Initial assessment should delineate the disturbances within the social systems pertinent to the request for service. Decisions about which social system is primarily involved and who should participate in the initial conference can determine the whole course of further assessment and intervention. These decisions often require extensive skilled exploratory telephone interactions with major members of the systems involved.

Effective social systems intervention is shaped by the intervener's ongoing appraisal of internal system conflicts in areas such as role, leadership, communication, and reinforcement. It is shaped, as well, by his assessment of the external stresses impinging on the system and the attempts by the system to cope with these stresses.

Ecological Precipitants of Systems Disturbances. In most instances, environmental stresses disturb the structure and function of the system by reactivating unresolved conflicts within it. A real or threatened separation in the primary social system of the identified patient was a major contributor to the request for service in 80 percent of patients at the Fort Logan Crisis Service. Work crises, sudden onset of medical illness, move or migration, death, financial difficulties, and pregnancy were also common.

Internal Precipitants of Systems Disturbances. Environmental precipitants often activate long-standing internal conflicts in a social organization. The conflicts may become so intense that they can no longer be handled by the system's routine coping mechanisms.

> A husband had been extremely dependent on his wife throughout their 15-year marriage, and the wife got a good deal of gratification from taking care of him. Both had strong, unexpressed fears of separation, which were intensified by the sudden death of the wife's father. The loss not only activated the couple's fears of separation, but also required actual separation when the wife left to attend the funeral. The resulting crisis brought the husband to psychiatric treatment with symptoms of depression.

Systems Coping Patterns. It is useful to get an initial picture of the coping mechanisms and the helping resources used by the system prior to contacting a mental health facility. Existing community personnel, such as ministers, neighbors, and friends, can often be involved productively in the process of intervention.[12]

A systems coping process involving labeling, scapegoating, and extrusion is an integral part of most requests for admission to a psychiatric hospital. At the point of admission the patient's family may communicate nonverbally: "There is no problem with us. The illness of the patient is the only problem." Admission without clarification of the pertinent family problem reinforces this viewpoint, and 2 weeks later family members may refuse involvement in family treatment.

Extrusive processes often provide valuable entry points into the systems disturbance. The pressure for extrusion can be used as a motivating force to bring the system together. The systems intervener, by skillfully clarifying and making explicit nonverbal extrusive themes, can then facilitate initial processes of systems change.

Psychiatric Illness Within Social Systems Disturbance: An Integrated Definition of the Problem to be Treated. The most important step in the assessment of clinical problems is the definition of the problem to be worked on in treatment. The hospitalized psychiatric patient tends to define the problem within the group of people with whom he lives and interacts outside the hospital, whereas the clinician defines the problem within the patient.[3]

The social systems model assumes that the individual with symptoms of psychiatric illness is a representative of one or more disturbed social systems which determine the psychiatric behavior of the identified patient; his illness behavior, in turn, may contribute to the disturbance. The social system assessor, therefore, focuses his attention on the structure and functioning of these social systems, and the assessment of the problems of individuals takes place within this framework.

Social Systems Intervention

Time and Place. Interactions with social organizations take place most effectively on the home ground of the system involved, such as the place of work, the classroom, or the home. Sessions begin at a predetermined time as soon as possible after the request for assistance. Specific time commitments, such as other appointments, are fed in at the beginning of the session. The process of the interaction then determines a natural ending point. Some sessions last 30 minutes, but most require at least an hour and one-half, and some may continue for 5 hours or more. One or two long sessions often can accomplish more than shorter sessions of regular outpatient therapy over an extended period.

Social System Membership. The usual procedure is to call together the main members of the system involved for a face-to-face meeting. However, several systems may be concerned in any one problem, and it may be useful either to call together the total membership of several systems in one session or to bring together all members of the primary social system and major representatives of other systems. Natural social systems usually have flexible, rather than permanent boundaries. A family may consist of two parents and three children in one session and may include grandparents in another. A neighbor may drop in and participate in a session. Intervention should follow these natural systems boundaries rather than following an artificial membership pattern presumed by the clinician.

Fred, a teen-ager, was referred from jail after narrowly missing his father with a rifle shot. Intervention focused on the primary social system comprising Fred, his brother, his parents, and, at times, his grandparents. Major representatives of other important social systems, rather than their total membership, were regular participants in the meetings in Fred's home, which focused on the marital problems of Fred's parents. The principal of the school from which Fred had been expelled three times for truancy and striking a teacher was a useful contributor to these sessions, along with a staff member of a mental health clinic who had initiated proceedings for Fred's transfer to a locked ward in a state hospital and Fred's parole officer.

Leadership. Because social systems intervention often involves complex and highly emotional interactions, we have found it preferable to include at least two skilled leaders in each session, one of whom is free to become involved in the process while the other can retain a broader perspective. These roles may be reversed later. In addition, two or more interveners can facilitate training by having reviews after each session in which they comment on each other's performances.

The Community Spokesman. The natural community spokesman, like the double in psychodrama, speaks for, and at times confronts, members of the system when they are experiencing difficulties in communicating. But, unlike the psychodrama double, the community spokesman plays this role for the individual or family in real life and is asked to participate in sessions on this basis.

A teen-age girl and her mother were in conflict over the girl's use of drugs and her repeated running away. We asked both the girl and the mother to bring spokesmen to the session who could effectively represent their viewpoints. The mother asked her mother to attend because the daughter had lived with her grandmother for a month and similar problems had emerged. The daughter asked a pregnant teen-age friend, who proved to be the most skillful intervener present. Her confrontation about the daughter's "plastic" behavior was the key to opening communication between mother and daughter.

Characteristics of Interveners. Our experience is that psychiatrists, psychologists, social workers, nurses, and psychiatric technicians or aides all can function as primary coordinators in social systems work. Our initial experience involving professional and nonprofessional natural community helpers, such as parole officers and neighbors, in social systems intervention suggests that a significant number of these individuals learn social systems techniques rapidly.

Professional training in mental health often results in the incorporation of a set of values and assumptions that interfere with effective social systems intervention. Prominent among these is the assumption that most problems can be defined within individuals. As a result, the untrained person with rich life experience and natural psychological sensitivity has several initial advantages over the professional. He has no firm set of assumptions and values that must be challenged and tends to be open to the obvious total systems disturbance as soon as he comes in contact with it. If the professionally trained person, however, is able to struggle through the first 6 to 12 months of confrontation with conflicting values, he is able to bring social systems work a greater depth of understanding and conceptualization than the untrained individual.

Techniques of Intervention

Face-to-Face Confrontation. Crisis resolution leading to growth consists of an immediate face-to-face meeting of all the members of the organization in crisis in the presence of one or more skilled, objective leaders who encourage open communication about the problems contributing to the crisis. We have found this technique to be broadly applicable to social systems intervention.[13]

Pace and Level of Feeling. Our experience suggests that the monitoring of the level of feeling and the pace of sessions should develop according to the values and defenses of the system, which are often very different from those of the clinician. Since the system is usually in a crisis, warm-up procedures are rarely necessary. As a general rule, we go as far and as fast as the system allows and make no presuppositions about what is too touchy to bring into the open. We have found that the system lets us know quite clearly, either overtly or covertly, when we have reached areas that are beyond its abilities to incorporate.

A family may be able to deal openly in a first session with a psychotic son's direct expression of incestuous feelings toward his mother. They may productively struggle with the father's feelings of jealousy, the mother's seductiveness toward the son, sexual problems between the parents, and the son's sexual inhibitions. This same family, however, might find it impossible to allow the father to cry or to express feelings of weakness. When we encounter resistance, our practice is to back off, to explore the touchy area carefully, and perhaps to pursue a different course.

Nonverbal Communication. The single most useful technique for social systems intervention, in our experience, is the ongoing monitoring and direct feedback to the system of nonverbal communication patterns.[14,15] Staying at the level of present nonverbal communication in the system often dramatically opens up emotion-laden sources of conflict.

Nonverbal themes or scripts representing the style of interaction in the system and the expected role of the helper often emerge clearly from the first telephone interaction, when it can be useful to respond in a way that contradicts the script.

A woman whose husband was driven to distraction by her hypochondriacal complaints said in her second or third telephone sentence that she really was not sure that I could help her. Instead of reassuring her that I could help, convincing her of my therapeutic power, and persuading her to participate in a therapeutic interaction, I agreed cheerfully that I, too, doubted that there was anything I could do to help her. This opened up for discussion the repetitive game in which both husband and therapist ended up as impotent helpers.

Special Techniques. The use of special techniques, such as psychodrama, depends on the personal style and preference of the intervener. For example, when a husband and wife are disagreeing heatedly but not communicating, doubling techniques might be applied to clarify their disagreement. It may be useful to interrupt the argument and to have the couple sit directly facing each other and say only complimentary things to each other for 2 minutes and then comment on the process. As is true of other techniques for effective social system intervention, methods must fit into the natural social structure of the system, rather than expecting the system to organize itself around the technique.[16]

The above principles are illustrated in the following case history:

Tom Parkes was referred because he was reported to be depressed, and the parole officer was afraid that he might commit a rape. Tom had spent 13 of his 36 years in prison, having been convicted at age 18 on five counts of aggravated rape. He had been on parole 5 years.

Initial assessment revealed that all his life Tom had been involved in a very stormy relationship with his mother. She was regarded as a domineering, controlling woman, and during the group psychotherapy that Tom had received in prison, she was identified as a major cause of his antisocial behavior. Tom was bitter about the way she controlled his life but resisted breaking off with her. Mrs. Parkes was described as a suspicious recluse, who never went out and who lived on only milk and orange juice. Tom was very concerned about his mother's health, but she seemed to almost enjoy presenting herself as a weakened, medically ill woman. She complained of sores on her scalp, anemia, and difficulty in walking.

Tom had a girl friend who apparently fit into his mother's mold. She was a "good girl" who evoked guilt and who was unavailable sexually. On the day of his last rape, he and his mother had shopped for a used car. The mother, who went with Tom at his request, had definite ideas about the kind of car Tom should buy. His ideas were the opposite, but finally he resentfully bought the car she liked. That evening Tom drove with his girl friend to a country lane and spent 2 hours trying to get her to have intercourse with him. He was extremely understanding of her refusal; he said he realized she was a good girl, and he was aware of no feelings of hostility toward her. Later he went cruising in his car and found a girl walking in downtown Denver. He put a rope around her neck and threatened her with a knife. He got her into the car, drove her to the same country lane, and raped her. He then had a long talk with her, took her for coffee, showed her his driver's license, and dropped her off.

Tom said that the greatest pleasure he derived during rape was at the moment he accosted a girl and she was totally helpless and in his power. It seemed especially striking to us that although Tom was sophisticated and perceptive about many things, he was incredibly naïve about the relationship between the rape and his interactions with his mother and his girl friend directly preceding it. We though that an obvious avenue to social system intervention would be the clarification of Tom's interactions with important women in his life. Tom's parole officer was a key community helping agent throughout this process.

Because of the mother's suspiciousness, it was necessary to use the same telephone signaling device that Tom used to get in touch with her, a process of allowing the phone to ring twice, hanging up, and immediately redialing. In our first telephone contact Tom's mother was extremely guarded and suspicious about my intentions. After long negotiations, she consented to come with Tom for a session. She was a well-made-up and not really very frail-looking, gray-haired lady who demanded to talk to me alone before she would commit herself to anything further. After we assured her that our conversation was not being recorded by a hidden microphone, we had a long talk interlaced with sanctimonious statements on her part about self-sacrifice and the meaning of life. While we were meeting, a psychiatric technician and the parole officer met with Tom. The major theme of their conference was helping Tom recognize situations in which he became angry at his mother.

When the mother and I joined Tom and the others, she said that she would do everything in her power to help her unfortunate son and his condition. Tom confronted her with the implied put-down, and an angry exchange ensued. In the following sessions, Tom and his mother became increasingly aware of the forces producing their nonverbal, angry interactions. Tom had failed repeatedly to meet his mother's high expectations of him. He became more aware of his need to keep her in a controlling, interfering role and then to scapegoat her as the source of all his difficulties. The mother, on the other hand, expressed relief that she could move from her accustomed role of assuming almost total responsibility for Tom to looking out more for her own welfare. It came out that Mrs. Parkes had been raped by her stepfather when she was a young woman. Tom's father had left her when Tom was quite young, and she was bitter because he had refused to help support her.

During one session, Mrs. Parkes raised her concern about how to express affection for her son without having her intentions confused with sexual interest. Some role-playing techniques were used, in the course of which the mother played the role of one of Tom's rape victims. At another point, Tom forcibly removed the parole officer from his position in front of the door when his mother sobbingly asked permission to leave the session. At the end of seven sessions, Tom seemed more in touch with his angry, hostile feelings toward his mother, his girl friend, and women in general and had moved toward being more assertive and independent in relation to his mother. At the same time, the mother gained some awareness of her hostility toward her son and of her legitimate frustrations at the way she was treated by men, including her son.

At this point, the sessions involving crisis unit staff stopped. The parole officer, who had participated in the training-centered review after each session continued meeting with Tom and his mother with crisis staff as consultants. They decided to include Tom's girl friend in their meetings. In the months that followed, Tom got very angry at his girl friend and stopped himself on the verge of raping her. She agreed to have sexual relations with him and did so, but without much enjoyment. They eventually developed a more satisfactory sexual relationship and got married, an event that Tom celebrated by sending me a cigar. To date, Tom has maintained a good work adjustment with recent promotion to managerial level. The parole officer reports that 18 months after intervention, there is no evidence to suggest that Tom has been involved in another rape.

REFERENCES

1. McPartland, T. S., and Richart, R. H.: Social and Clinical Outcomes of Psychiatric Treatment. Arch. Gen. Psychiat. (Chicago) 14:179-184, 1966.
2. Ellsworth, R., Foster, L., Childers, B., Arthur, G., and Kroeker, D.: Hospital and Community Adjustment as Perceived by Psychiatric Patients, Their Families and Staff. J. Consult. Clin. Psychol. 32(suppl.):5, 2, 1968.
3. Polak, P.: Patterns of Discord: Goals of Patients, Therapists, and Community Members. Arch. Gen. Psychiat. (Chicago) 23:277-283, 1970.
4. Polak, P.: The Irrelevance of Hospital Treatment to the Patient's Social System. Hosp. Community Psychiat. 22(8):43-44, 1971.
5. Anderson, M., Polak, P., Grace, D., and Lee, A.: Treatment Goals for Patients from Patients, Their Families, and Staff. J. Fort Logan Ment. Health Cent. 3:101-115, 1965.
6. Polak, P.: The Crisis of Admission. Soc. Psychiat. 2:150-157, 1967.
7. Davidites, Rose Marie: A Social Systems Approach to Deviant Behavior. Amer. J. Nurs. 71(8):1588-1589, 1971.
8. Jones, M.: Beyond the Therapeutic Community: Social Learning and Social Psychiatry. New Haven, Conn., Yale University Press, 1968.
9. Kraft, A.: The Therapeutic Community. In: Arieti, S. (Ed.), American Handbook of Psychiatry, Vol. 3. New York, Basic Books, Inc., 1966, pp. 542-551.
10. Tyhurst, J. S.: The Role of Transition States Including Disaster in Mental Illness: Symposium on Preventive and Social Psychiatry. Walter Reed, Army Institute of Research & National Research Council, U.S. Government Printing Office, 1957, pp. 142-167.
11. Lindemann, E.: Symptomatology and Management of Acute Grief. Amer. J. Psychiat. 101:141-148, 1944.
12. Caplan, G.: Principles of Preventive Psychiatry. London, Tavistock Publications, Ltd., 1964.
13. Jones, M., and Polak, P.: Crisis and Confrontation. Brit. J. Psychiat. 114:169-174, 1968.
14. Fish, L.: Social Systems Treatment Techniques. Hosp. Community Psychiat. 22(8):252-255, 1971.
15. Eisler, R.: Crisis Intervention in the Family of a Firesetter. To be published in Psychotherapy: Theory, Research and Practice.
16. Polak, P.: Social Systems Intervention. Arch. Gen. Psychiat. (Chicago) 25:110-117, 1971.

Home Visiting: An Aid to Psychiatric Treatment in Black Urban Ghettos

by John N. Chappel, M.D., and Robert S. Daniels, M.D.

Developments in community psychiatry during the past decade reflect increased interest in extending the locus of treatment from office and hospital to home and community. Centers reporting on the use of psychiatric home visits are enthusiastic about the technique as an adjunct to therapy.[1,2] Studies in Boston and California report over 70 percent of psychiatrists in practice making one or more home visits a year.[3,4]

The experiences reported in this chapter took place on the south side of Chicago over a period of 3 years. Early data were gained during a 3-month study of hospitalized patients from the urban community of Woodlawn.[5] This community is predominantly black and could be described as an urban slum, with high rates in most indices of social disorganization.

The authors have been involved with two psychiatric treatment programs which continue to utilize home visits. The Woodlawn Mental Health Center conducts an active aftercare program for patients with acute and chronic emotional disturbances. This program includes home visiting by psychiatrists and community mental health workers. The latter group do most of the visiting, but when difficult treatment problems are encountered, psychiatric home visits have been found valuable. The second resource is the Illinois Drug Abuse Program, which provides treatment for over 2000 narcotics addicts in the Chicago area. Home visiting by psychiatrists, nurses, and addiction specialists is used both for crisis intervention and as part of ongoing treatment.

Common Objections to Home Visiting

A number of barriers block the acceptance of home visiting by psychiatrists as a tool for improving treatment. Lip service may be paid to potential value, but there is little evidence that home visiting occupies an important role in psychiatric training or practice. The following objections are frequently raised:

1. Home visiting is expensive in terms of both time and money.
2. Home visiting may be difficult and dangerous, especially in ghetto slums.
3. Home visiting may interfere with treatment by providing secondary gain which leads to acting out or excessive dependence.
4. Home visiting may impose a burden on family and community by keeping an emotionally ill person at home.
5. Home visiting is not a function for psychiatrists but is more appropriately the role of nurses, social workers, or other mental health workers.

We feel that many of these objections are not always valid and may often reflect internal resistance more than external reality. The economics of home visiting should be viewed in the context of the cost of hospitalization. Mickle[2] states that home visits may prevent hospitalization. In other cases, time may actually be saved with patients who are very difficult to evaluate in the office.[1] The psychiatrist tends to be more active in the patient's home and the patient and his family are less defensive.[2]

The dangers facing psychiatrists in black urban ghettos do not appear great. No episodes of harm or violence have been reported in the literature or experienced by the authors, even in periods of civil unrest. The cost in psychic energy is offset by the change of pace which can provide an effective antidote for the loneliness which characterizes individual psychotherapy.

There is no convincing evidence that patients abuse home visits or are damaged by them. Benefit to the patient-therapist relationship is most evident with lower-socioeconomic-class patients.[6] Rather than leading to the development of dependence, the home visit often gives rise to a sense of relief that the therapist is human and cares enough to extend himself. Interpretation of behavior and limit setting can be effective safeguards against patient abuse.

Maintaining a patient in his home at any cost is not a major treatment goal. Home visiting should be evaluated in terms of its contribution to improved function, decreased symptomatic disturbance, and diminished stress for the family and community. Our experience has been that home visiting can be a source of both education and support for the patient's family. Confidence in the therapist may be increased, thus enhancing his ability to alter environmental and family forces affecting the patient.

The main reason for home visiting by the psychiatrist is that this activity can be a potent force in facilitating therapy and establishing a therapeutic alliance. Behrens[6] states that even one brief home visit helps establish rapport and avoids communication difficulties in the treatment of lower-socioeconomic-class patients. The experience in the home increases the psychiatrist's knowledge of the patient and his awareness of the nonverbal interactions that characterize the family dynamics.

Indications for Home Visiting

1. Crises in treatment which result in a plea for help from the family, especially if the alternative appears to be commitment, hospitalization, or imprisonment.
2. Reluctance of the patient to continue treatment, diminishing motivation, or absence from treatment in the face of a clearly continuing need for help.
3. Relapses in the course of treatment which cannot be understood in the context of the patient-therapist relationship.
4. Difficulty in communicating with or understanding the patient.
5. Transfer of a patient from one treatment modality to another, especially following discharge from hospital to an outpatient aftercare program.
6. Teaching and supervision of psychiatry residents or medical students on a treatment team.

When the indications are present and a decision has been made to visit a patient's home, the visit will be found to fall into two phases. Each phase has its own characteristics and challenges.

The Community Phase

Venturing into an urban ghetto frequently arouses anxiety in the visitor. Familiarity with the community, its residents, and others working there can do much to allay unsettling anxiety. Trust in the neighborhood grapevine and the presence of a companion known in the community help dull hackle-raising fantasy of a bullet in the back of the head. A sense of purpose and belief in the value of the visit helps raise flagging motivation.

Planning. Prearranged visits are frequently disappointing. Our experience parallels that of Meyer et al.,[7] who found that, even with patient preparation and agreement, it was not unusual to find no one home at the scheduled time. Permission for the visit is best obtained in person at the door of the home, since prior requests are often turned down. Anxiety levels and resistance to home visits may be even higher in the visited than in the visitor. One man, after learning that a visit was planned for later in the week, went so far as to move out of his hotel room without leaving a forwarding address.

The most successful time for finding ghetto dwellers at home has been late afternoon or Saturday morning. Once the visitor and his purpose have been made clear, even the most suspicious persons will usually grant permission for the visit. In every instance the authors have been admitted to patients' homes.

Attitude of the Visitor in the Community. The best protection for a visitor may be an open willingness to identify himself. We do not hesitate to ask for help from people in the street. This can be done without revealing damaging information about the patient. We have yet to hear objections or to receive complaints following home visits from a psychiatrist.

Locating the Home. In deteriorating urban areas there may be no address numbers on buildings, mailboxes without names, and an absence of numbers on apartment doors. Persistent door knocking, seeking out and greeting the janitor, or stopping people may be required to locate the patient's place of residence.

In our experience ghetto dwellers with mental illness are characterized by a striking degree of social isolation. Alienation and hopelessness characterize the lives of many of our patients. Social distance seems to be part of the slum way of life. Frequently people do not know their neighbors in the next apartment.

The following case illustrates isolation, extensive pathology, and the value of persistence in pursuing community contacts.

Case 1. Mr. R. R., age 33, was a musician who had been unable to work at his profession for three years, since his marriage ended in divorce. Mrs. R., his ex-wife, had him committed when he demanded money from her, refused to leave her apartment, and lay down on the floor, making threats and delusional comments.

Mr. R. had been in intermittent treatment as an outpatient for several years. During these contacts almost nothing was learned of his life circumstances. He had sought help because he hallucinated that his skin was changing from brown to orange and because he suffered from impotence. On no occasion would he reveal his address and telephone number.

Throughout the interview in the hospital Mr. R. was suspicious and guarded. He was insistent in his wishes that the psychiatrist talk to no one about him. The psychiatrist did not agree and stressed the importance of finding better ways to deal with his problems, since past methods had not worked well.

Telephone contact with Mrs. R. led to a home visit with Mr. R.'s mother. This elderly, withdrawn woman lived alone in a small room in an old apartment building. Her husband had died shortly after the birth of Mr. R., her youngest child. The three children had been sent to a foster home when the patient was 14 months old. Contact between the mother and the children was intermittent and stormy. A few years previously the middle child, a daughter, had stabbed her mother.

The daughter had recently been admitted to Manteno State Hospital and turned out to be Mrs. K. S., another patient in the clinic, whom the psychiatrist had been unable to contact because of an incorrect address. A home visit with Mrs. S. revealed that Mr. R. had been both intelligent and talented. He had graduated in the top ten of his high school class and had shown no sign of emotional problems until he married. Mrs. S. blamed her brother's wife for his sexual problems. She did not feel that she could be of any help to her brother but expressed an interest in visiting him in the hospital. Finally, she promised to persuade him to join the aftercare program where both of them could obtain medication and group therapy.

The home visits revealed extensive family pathology that had not been evident during the long period when the patient was in outpatient treatment.

198 CURRENT PSYCHIATRIC THERAPIES: 1972

The family, which had previously shown no obvious interest, now agreed that help was necessary. The cooperative attitude displayed in the homes was in marked contrast to the guarded suspiciousness shown in the hospital.

The Home Phase

Once identification has been made, and double or triple locks have been opened, the second phase of the visit begins. Do not expect coffee or social amenities. There is no automatic acceptance of the psychiatrist. Deep suspicion is likely to be present regarding his motivation and interest in the patient.

Relate to the Male of the Family. The Moynihan report on the Negro family in America emphasized the absence of a man in the home and the relatively better education and earning power of women. It is our impression that the black man's current role in the family is more important than is usually apparent. Two patterns tend to emerge. Either the man expects to be avoided or ignored if he is not the patient or, less frequently, he will be authoritative, dominant, and even militant. In either case, the man's cooperation and understanding are important both to the success of treatment of family members and to support the existing family structure.

Be Alert to the Patient's Agenda. In addition to the therapist's agenda for the visit, he must be sensitive to the patient's expectations. Mutual definition of the objectives and purposes of treatment can do much to facilitate further treatment. Avoiding implied promises and dealing with hidden expectations of ongoing treatment in the home will often prevent later difficulties.

The following case illustrates both hidden agendas and hidden pathology. Hospitalization had been used for years to obscure family needs. When the needs of each family member were recognized, it became possible to terminate hospitalization without forcing the patient to return home. Appropriate help was also obtained for other individuals within the family.

Case 2. Mr. C. D., age 49, had been in the state hospital for 18 years. During most of this time he had been a "good" patient. When interviewed, his manner was bland and he displayed virtually no affect. The hospital staff felt that he had been ready for discharge for some time. They were frustrated by their inability to get Mrs. D. to come in and discuss the possibility of her husband's discharge.

Mrs. D. was visited in her apartment in a public housing project. She was an attractive, cooperative, hospitable woman who kept her home clean and well furnished. While her husband had been hospitalized she had raised the three children by herself and supported them by working as a practical nurse in a local hospital. In addition, she had taken night classes and correspondence courses, attaining the equivalent of three years of college education. It had been her practice to take any civil service examination for which she was eligible.

One year before the visit she had been appointed as a truant officer. This work was done during the day in the same area in which she lived. Her two jobs created a problem in that she made too much money and had to move out of the housing project.

In this apparently benign setting the strange tale of the children was revealed. The oldest son, age 23, was a patient in Manteno State Hospital. He had been discharged from the Army the previous summer for psychiatric reasons. One month before the home visit her younger son, age 21, had been shot in a subway station where he was accused of having attempted to rape a woman. The next night the oldest son tried to get into bed with his mother. She became quite upset at this and had him committed.

The younger son was still in jail awaiting psychiatric evaluation. He had suffered from severe eczema as a child and was always depressed. Throughout adolescence he had often been in trouble and had said several times that he would die early. Most of his crimes were clumsily performed, and he was almost always caught.

The daughter, age 18, was born four weeks after her father was committed to Manteno. She had dropped out of school in grade nine and now had an illegitimate child. Eighteen months before the home visit she began breaking up everything made of glass in the apartment. She was admitted to a psychiatric ward for one week. She then left home, and there had been no repetition of the destructive behavior.

Mrs. D. made it plain that she did not want any of her family living with her, especially her husband. She felt that she had outgrown him and did not want him discharged in her care. He could live with other members of his own family. Her hope was to remarry and start a new life.

As a result of the home visit a family session was held at the hospital. Mrs. D. looked as though she had stepped out of a fashion magazine. The words she spoke to her son expressed care and concern, but her nonverbal communication was rejecting. Mr. D. remained a passive spectator and seemed oblivious to what was going on around him. Arrangements were made for Mr. D. to be discharged to live with a relative. The son returned home with his mother and was referred to an aftercare program where he could receive medication and psychotherapy.

Open All Senses. The combination of visual, auditory, olfactory, tactile, and emotional sensations provides a new context for communication with the patient. Experiencing firsthand the environment of the ghetto dweller can add another dimension to understanding his life stress. Nonverbal communication may be even more important than what is verbally offered. Do not hesitate to move around the house if invited or indicated by circumstances. Strengths in the form of alliances and support may become evident in a way that is rarely appreciated when the patient comes to a clinic or office.

It may be possible to increase the strength of family support available to the patient. The therapist may serve as a source of education and support for members of the family. Home visiting appears to increase the family's confidence in the therapist and to enhance his ability to alter environmental and social forces affecting the patient. In addition, the home experience increases the psychiatrist's knowledge of the patient and his awareness of the nonverbal interactions that characterize the family dynamics. These opportunities are often missed in the hospital or clinic. Either important family members do not come to the institution or, when they do, they are too overwhelmed, inhibited, or irritated to ask the questions or express the feelings that concern them the most.

Use of a Companion. We have been impressed with the advantages of visiting with a paraprofessional colleague, such as a community mental health worker or addiction counselor who is familiar with the community. Communication is facilitated between patient, family, and therapist with less chance of mutual misunderstanding. In our experience the presence of a companion is particularly useful in developing a working relationship with paranoid or violent patients.

On two dramatic occasions men with guns had terrified their peers and family. Home visits were undertaken with a black male paraprofessional. In each case the crisis was relieved. Both men were found to be desperate. They had hoped to be killed, hurt badly, or incarcerated. This behavior was understood as a means of inflicting injury on people whom they thought no longer cared about them and also as a way of relieving guilt and shame. A profound loss of self-esteem related to job failure was present in each man. During the course of the visits violent threats dissolved into tears. Both incarceration and hospitalization were avoided. With over a year of follow-up in each case there has been no repetition of violent behavior. One of the men has become a youth counselor and has enrolled in a university mental health career program.

Conclusion

Controlled studies will be necessary to evaluate critically the role of psychiatric home visits in the treatment of black ghetto residents. Our experiences to date, however, offer some evidence that the advantages gained outweigh the disadvantages. On the basis of our experience we find support for the following statements:

1. Psychiatric home visiting is both possible and safe in a black urban ghetto.
2. Home visiting can be effective in bridging the isolation, alienation, and hopelessness found in many ghetto patients.
3. Home visiting can enlist important treatment support from family members and friends not usually encountered in clinic or office settings.
4. Home visiting can be helpful in treating violent or paranoid patients and preventing acting out which disrupts treatment and requires hospitalization or incarceration.
5. Home visiting provides an effective nonverbal way of bridging social and cultural gaps which interfere with the development of a treatment relationship between patient and therapist. The latent language of the visit provides a basis for trust and invites the patient to participate actively in treatment.

Many black ghetto residents feel that the institutions serving the slums are insensitive to the real needs of the people. The riots, demonstrations, and civil rights protests of recent years make it plain that black and white Americans do not understand each other and mistrust each other's motives. Visits by a white professional into a black home can help increase understanding and begin to arouse interest in addition to achieving other treatment goals.

Large segments of inner-city populations are not served by psychiatric outpatient programs. Many symptomatic individuals do not actively seek treatment but may respond well once they are involved in therapy. Programs serving urban communities must find new ways to reach this apparently unmotivated, isolated, but needy population. Home visiting provides one way of achieving such a goal.

Acknowledgments

The authors acknowledge with gratitude the helpful comments and suggestions of Dr. George Meyer, Professor of Psychiatry, University of Texas, San Antonio, and Dr. Charles Wilkinson, Professor of Psychiatry, University of Missouri, Kansas City.

REFERENCES

1. Freeman, R. D.: The Home Visit in Child Psychiatry. J. Amer. Child Psychiat. 6:279-293, 1967.
2. Mickle, J. C.: Psychiatric Home Visits. Arch. Gen. Psychiat. (Chicago) 9:379-383, 1963.
3. Brown, B. S.: Home Visiting by Psychiatrists. Arch. Gen. Psychiat. (Chicago) 7:98-107, 1962.
4. Meyer, R. E., Schieff, L. F., and Becker, A.: The Home Treatment of Psychotic Patients: An Analysis of 154 Cases. Amer. J. Psychiat. 123:1430-1438, 1967.
5. Chappel, J. N., and Daniels, R. S.: Home Visiting in a Black Urban Community. Amer. J. Psychiat. 126:1455-1460, 1970.
6. Behrens, M. I.: Brief Home Visits by the Clinic Therapist in the Treatment of Lower-Class Patients. Amer. J. Psychiat. 124:127-131, 1967.
7. Meyer, G., Margolis, P., and Daniels, R.: Hospital Discharges Against Medical Advice. II. Outcome. Arch. Gen. Psychiat. (Chicago) 8:41-49, 1963.

A Psychiatric Program for the Deaf

by John D. Rainer, M.D., and Kenneth Z. Altshuler, M.D.

Many real and presumed difficulties previously stood in the way of providing psychiatric evaluation and treatment of persons profoundly deaf since birth or early childhood. In 1955, to satisfy the great unmet needs for such psychiatric facilities, to realize the many theoretical, clinical, and social gains to be derived from them, and to overcome the despair and neglect which had characterized this field, New York State inaugurated the first stage of a mental health program for the deaf.[1] This program has since developed into a comprehensive set of services for prevention, treatment, and rehabilitation.[2]

Previously, the pathways to an understanding of psychiatric symptoms and to the development and availability of treatment were blocked by formidable obstacles of communication. There were probably some more subtle bases for avoiding the problem as well: the soundless world of the deaf is unconsciously equated, by many persons, with lifelessness, with impenetrability, and with hopelessness regarding vital human contacts. Today, with the hindsight of 15 years, this attitude seems quite remote to those of us who have been associated with the deaf for that period of time. Everyone connected with the program has felt a fascination and devotion in spite of the many frustrations. This strongly positive investment may be caused by the inherent interest of the work, or the challenge of doing the seemingly impossible; by the gratification of success, or some special emotion and satisfaction in reaching the deaf. In any case, we have seen this reaction over the years among psychiatrists from many parts of the country and all over the world, and it bodes well for the extension of such work in the future.

The Deaf as a Population

Deafness is defined in the present context as a hearing loss from birth or early childhood, rendering a person incapable of substantial auditory contact with the environment. Occurring in about one person per thousand of the general population, deafness is associated with a relatively low but increasing marriage rate and a relatively high divorce rate. Over 90 percent of deaf persons marry other deaf persons. With about half of deafness exogenous (maternal rubella, meningitis in infancy, etc.), and about half hereditary (mostly recessive), only 10 percent overall of the children of deaf parents are also deaf. Conversely, most deaf children are born to and raised by hearing parents.

Deaf youngsters, if picked up early enough, are often given special preschool education and then enrolled in schools for the deaf, day or residential, or in day classes in regular schools. Parents on their part, however, can seldom find the support and guidance they need in dealing with their own emotional reactions to having a deaf child.

Socially, deaf people have formed associations, theater groups, athletic competitions, all on a worldwide basis; a liberal arts college (Gallaudet College, Washington), a technical institute (National Technical Institute for the Deaf, Rochester), and junior colleges provide higher education, and, though still relatively few, more and more deaf persons are achieving highly skilled or professional status.

A controversy, as yet largely unreconciled, persists between the exponents of strictly oral communication (lip reading and use of voice) and those advocating the combined use of oral and manual methods (above plus sign language and/or finger spelling). Whether early exposure to manual techniques makes it easier or more difficult to acquire the oral skills is unfortunately still the subject more of rancorous debate than of controlled experiment. In psychiatric work with deaf adults it is necessary to accommodate to every patient's means of communication, and therefore to become proficient by instruction and practice in manual language. Experience has shown that with daily use, a basic working vocabulary can be acquired in about 6 months. Interpreters, useful in many contacts with the deaf, are not best suited to the requirements of psychiatric interchange.

A general survey of the deaf population would reveal, in brief, a group handicapped by poor language ability, making slow progress toward social and self-acceptance and educational and vocational opportunity, but with generally a poor preparation for family living and underachieving patterns both in school and in work.

Character Traits and Symptoms

Psychiatric treatment methods have evolved out of some of the typical, possibly intrinsic, personality problems of the deaf, out of the special communication media used, and out of the social environments peculiar to the deaf as a handicapped and a minority group. Before we discuss methods and problems of therapy in various settings, some words regarding personality development and psychiatric disorder in the deaf are in place.[3]

During the early years of operation of our pilot clinic for the deaf, there was opportunity to see at firsthand some of the particular kinds of maladjustment and psychopathology in this group. In character there was noted a lack of empathy, a diminished understanding and regard for the feelings of other people, a lessened awareness of the impact of one's own behavior on other people, and the tendency toward impulsive actions with limited control and constraint. One corollary of the latter trait is that rage lies close to the surface rather than becoming internalized, and indeed little or no retarded depressive symptomatology was noted.[4] Paranoid symptoms and projective mechanisms were seen, but were not universal, and basically were no more prevalent than among hearing groups. Organized obsessional mechanisms were rare. The most prevalent diagnosis among nonpsychotic adult patients was passive-aggressive personality disorder.

Whether these character traits and symptom patterns are related to absence of verbal language per se, or to the lack of parent-child communication, relatedness, and interaction in the early years, is still a moot question. To put it another way, is it in language itself or in the closeness of contact which language brings that the clue to some of the character traits noted is to be found? Associational pathways may be different for the deaf child with diminished verbal thinking, and the altered language matrix in turn may alter the quality of experience. Poor abstraction ability may make it harder to rationalize, to generalize, and to siphon off emergency emotions—in short, to move from primary-process to secondary-process thought.

There is experimental evidence, nevertheless, that the deaf youngster is in no way intrinsically incapable of logical thought despite the lack of verbal proficiency.[5] Many persons have noted similarities between the deaf child and the culturally deprived child, and deafness may indeed be used as a special instance for the study of this large-scale general social problem. An extreme example is represented by a category of patients we have seen among our adolescents and adults which we have termed the primitive personality—a pervading social and cognitive immaturity found in some deaf persons who have had no communication at home at all, having been raised on the periphery of the family or by parents largely absent or themselves psychotic.

Psychotic Illness

Turning to psychotic, and particularly hospitalized, illness in the deaf, an important task of the mental health program during its entire development has been to study deaf patients in the various state institutions. In the deaf, psychiatric diagnosis is necessarily prolonged. The manual language used by many deaf persons is often only an approximation of the spoken word, with meanings open to subjective interpretation. Poor grammatical structure, exaggerated in manual communication, may mask or mimic a subtle disorder of thought. Idiomatic differences between spoken language and signing and a tendency to respond in concrete terms, so common among the deaf, further complicate the task.

In communicating nuances and emotional context, facial expressions and bodily gestures play a greater role in manual language than in normal speech. With this type of affective accentuation, the emotional expressivity of the deaf schizophrenic patient, for example, takes on an air of vitality and depth. Then, too, because of the intimate relation between ideational content and its gestural communication, dissociation of idea and affect, or incongruity between one and the other, is rare in all but the most poorly integrated patients. Prolonged observation is usually required to uncover clues such as slight but persistent inappropriateness of mood, defects of attention span, or hints of autistic thinking.

In surveying the state hospitals, the distribution of mental disorder in deaf and hearing patients at the start of our program showed some important differences. With relation to the total population, about twice as many deaf patients as hearing ones were hospital residents, but much of this excess was due to longer stay in the hospital because of blocks to diagnosis, treatment, and rehabilitation. Schizophrenia was about as common as in the hearing, with no excess of paranoid cases; mental deficiency often accompanied psychosis in organically caused deafness; retinitis pigmentosa replaced alcoholism as the most common organic syndrome, and retarded depression was notably rare as a symptom in both cycloid and involutional psychoses.

Inpatient Services

Since 1963, a unique psychiatric ward for the deaf has treated some 200 inpatients, male and female. The facility, the first of its kind, was designed to house 30 patients, 15 males and 15 females, and provide a staff that was professionally skilled and conversant with manual language. It is located in a specially altered section of Rockland State Hospital about 20 miles from New York City. Functioning as an intensive-treatment unit, it requires a large staff-to-patient ratio. Referrals are made by community agencies, private individuals, and schools, as well as for transfer from other state hospitals. Treatment includes psychotherapy, drug and somatic therapies, and a favorable ward milieu. Adjunctive treatments include occupational and recreational therapy, individual instruction in the "three r's," rehabilitation counseling with prevocational experience in the hospital, and social activities organized with the help of volunteers. A group therapy program conducted by the psychiatric staff with the use of the manual language and enhanced by videotape playback has proved to be an important vehicle to supplement individual treatment.

During the first pilot years of this inpatient program it was possible to discharge close to 50 percent of the patients over 25 years of age and 25 percent of the young adult group. Among those discharged were patients who had spent from 20 to 25 years in other hospitals and were able to be placed on convalescent care within months after their transfer. At the end of a 3-year demonstration period, the ward for the deaf plus the existing outpatient service was incorporated into the regular program of the New York State Department of Mental Hygiene and has served as a model for a number of similar programs subsequently begun in other parts of the United States and of the world. In the north of England, Denmark and Eldridge,[6] encountering similar problems of diagnosis and classification, have established a 26-bed inpatient unit for deaf patients at Whittingham Hospital and outpatient clinics both in Manchester and in London. Programs in Scandinavia include a Danish hospital where Remvig has treated 31 patients over a period of 6 years in a centralized unit[7]; in Norway, Basilier[8] works closely with patients at a mental hospital as well as at a special school for emotionally disturbed deaf children and adolescents. In this country a number of psychiatric services have been developed including those by Grinker and Vernon at Michael Reese Hospital in Chicago,[9] by Robinson at St. Elizabeth's Hospital in Washington, and by Schlesinger at the Langley Porter Clinic in San Francisco.[10]

Methods of Therapy

Psychotherapy with the deaf may be characterized according to its mode (individual or group), its technique of communication (manual or oral) with the resulting difficulties of interpretation and understanding, and its goal (personality change, symptom removal, or encouragement and support). The therapist may often be cast into the role of good provider, who is depended upon for specific help and advice in difficult problems and decisions. The childhood isolation, sheltered school years, and conceptual concreteness of many deaf persons tend to foster such expectations and much effective therapy can be done in this context. Self-esteem and daily functioning can be improved by suggesting environmental changes and encouraging independence of action and breakthrough of isolation. With some patients, their greater literacy, psychological sensitivity, or creative imagination makes it possible to engage in a more cooperative search for insight and personality release; in such cases, the pictorial imagery of the sign language, in conversation and in dream reporting, may actually be used to uncover important emotional associations.

The social isolation and lack of empathy of many deaf adolescents and adults, patterns of nonawareness of others, and noncooperation can be effectively attacked in group therapy. By noting the behavior and reactions of others, the group members can achieve a greater degree of objectivity about themselves, learn concepts and techniques of cooperation, and achieve greater social maturity. The therapist may draw the group's attention to discrepancies between aims and actions, between actions and results, and between applications of the golden rule to oneself and to others; in this process, he must have respect for the conceptual limitations and the impulsivity-immaturity constellation of his patients. In group treatment, patients have been able to yield some of their distorted perceptions, and with a sense of group identity has come the first empathic interest ever experienced by some of these estranged, conceptually limited, and personally isolated individuals.

Pharmacotherapy as an adjunct or principal method of treatment plays its usual role, with most deaf patients being quite willing to take the drugs and tolerant of high doses of phenothiazines.

Preventive Psychiatry

The establishment of therapeutic services made evident the need for expansion of the New York State program into the areas of preventive psychiatry and rehabilitation.[11]

It had been clear throughout the program that a good many of the problems seen in adolescents and adults could be traced back at least to the school years, which generally offer the first chance for persons outside the family to note any signs of early disorder. In our initial survey, we found that deaf criminals and offenders had consistently shown a history of behavior or difficulty while in school, and many clinic referrals from schools had been made for sexual problems, stealing, and other symptoms of disturbed personality. A consulting relationship with a school for the deaf was established, and this experience uncovered a large but unmet need for individual and group counseling for deaf students and for assisting them in developing concepts of responsibility and feelings of concern for others. There was also a paucity of psychiatric guidance for teachers, cottage parents, and other staff to help them in encouraging healthy identifications, attitudes, and development in their charges. And certainly the role of the parents, even for the child who spends most of his week in a residential school—perhaps particularly for this child—was insufficiently emphasized. Parents had little chance to voice their common problems with their children, as well as their own feelings of shame and guilt, resulting in various combinations of rejection and overprotection.

For these reasons, individual consultations at the school were supplemented by meetings with the teachers and house parents, both individually and in groups. In addition, meetings with adolescent student groups, as with the hospital patients described earlier, were undertaken to enhance their abilities to observe themselves and others, to give them a framework in which to define the consequences of their own behavior, to deepen their conceptual grasp and sense of mutual interest and responsibility, and to foster better identification with the rules and roles of sexual and family behavior. Videotape recording has provided instant playback for objective self-observation. Finally, group sessions with parents of students, both deaf and hearing parents of younger children as well as those of full-grown adolescents, have helped to ferret out many of their guilts, fears, denials—all resistances to a healthy stance with respect to their children—and helped them realize that the others shared their difficulties.

Rehabilitation

Effective as treatment can be when provided by a team familiar with the language, the sociology, and the personality characteristics of the deaf, persistent bottlenecks can block a program when community agencies are not available to shelter and receive patients who are ready for referral. In the New York State program, the addition of a vocational rehabilitation counselor and the establishment of better liaison with state vocational rehabilitation agencies and outside training facilities have made it possible to consider discharge plans for inpatients early in their hospital stay. At the same time, the recruitment of a trained social worker and a teacher has paved the way for the patients' more effective return to the community. All these services are available to outpatients and those in aftercare as well.

A major step in the rehabilitation program was the establishment of a close working relationship with Fountain House, a halfway house in New York City serving former psychiatric patients, whereby its services were extended to the deaf. With the aid of a special counselor to coordinate the work with deaf patients, the following programs were made available: intramural work in the kitchen, clerical department, and housekeeping units, social programs and recreational activities, a transitional employment program with placement in community industries and stores, and an apartment program establishing independent living arrangements. Some of the patients have been able to begin these activities while still in the hospital.

Further Extension of Services

Psychiatric treatment of the deaf as it developed in New York State has come to embody the elements of a comprehensive and sequential set of psychiatric services. These services started basically from a research interest and developed by their own momentum; as the needs became evident, programs were designed to fit them, and without deliberate intent the project came to meet most of the requirements for a community mental health facility. As summarized at a conference of psychiatrists for the deaf,[12] a pragmatically oriented program of prevention, treatment, and rehabilitation will function in various ways at appropriate stages: support and education for the parents of deaf infants; instructional methods in early grades based on knowledge of emotional development and concept formation; experience in socialization and group adjustment provided by teachers, dormitory counselors, and school guidance persons; trouble shooting, crisis intervention, and individual therapy when psychiatric problems arise; hospitalization, aftercare, and rehabilitation; public awareness of the deaf, their achievements and special needs. In 1968, a group of mental health professionals in various disciplines—rehabilitation workers, psychologists, social workers, educators, audiologists, speech pathologists, and clergymen—defined their roles in this scheme at a national conference whose report[13] provides many details regarding the integrated approach to mental health care for the deaf.

Besides the extension of the kind of treatment program described here to other areas of the country, there are new programs that have to be started to fulfill needs as yet unmet.[14] Many of these are in the area of child psychiatry. Preventive efforts should be extended to the very young deaf child. Research has to be planned into the interactions within the family during the first year or two of his life, and guidelines for parents must be developed and disseminated. Better use of psychiatrists must be made in the schools, with child psychiatrists becoming more interested in some of the problems of the deaf child. Finally, special schools for emotionally disturbed deaf children need to be established, where children who cannot remain in the ordinary classroom may be temporarily transferred for special management and treatment. Facilities for the care of the deaf mentally retarded, provision for marriage counseling, and better guidelines to courts and law enforcement agencies are among the other directions in which psychiatric understanding may most beneficially proceed. For all these, many new professionals are sorely needed to explore the considerable merits of this long-overlooked but richly rewarding psychiatric byway.

REFERENCES

1. Rainer, J. D., Altshuler, K. Z., and Kallmann, F. J.: Family and Mental Health Problems in a Deaf Population, 2nd ed. Springfield, Ill., Charles C Thomas, Publisher, 1969.
2. Rainer, J. D., and Altshuler, K. Z.: Comprehensive Mental Health Services for the Deaf. New York, New York State Psychiatric Institute, 1966.
3. Altshuler, K. Z.: Studies of the Deaf: Relevance to Psychiatric Theory. Amer. J. Psychiat. 127:1521-1526, 1971.
4. Altshuler, K. Z.: Personality Traits and Depressive Symptoms in the Deaf. In: Wortis, J. (Ed.), Recent Advances in Biological Psychiatry, Vol. VI. New York, Plenum Press, 1963, pp. 63-73.
5. Furth, H. G.: Thinking Without Language: Psychological Implications of Deafness. New York, Free Press, 1966.
6. Denmark, J. C., and Eldridge, R. W.: Psychiatric Services for the Deaf. Lancet 2:259-262, 1969.
7. Remvig, J.: Deaf-Mutism and Psychiatry. Acta Psychiat. Scand. (Suppl 210), Copenhagen, Munksgaard, 1969.
8. Basilier, T.: Commentary on the Mental Health Needs of Deaf People. In: Lloyd, G. T. (Ed.), International Research Seminar on the Vocational Rehabilitation of Deaf Persons. U.S. Social and Rehabilitation Service, 1968, pp. 372-376.
9. Grinker, R.: Psychiatric Diagnosis, Therapy and Research on the Psychotic Deaf. Final Report Project RD 2407-S. U.S. Social and Rehabilitation Service, 1969.
10. Schlesinger, H. S., and Meadow, K. P.: Deafness and Mental Health: A Developmental Approach, Final Report, Project RD 2835-S. Langley Porter Neuropsychiatric Institute, 1971; also University of California Press (in press).

11. Rainer, J. D., and Altshuler, K. Z. (Eds.): Expanded Mental Health Care for the Deaf: Rehabilitation and Prevention. Final Report Project RD 2128-S. U.S. Social and Rehabilitation Service, 1970.
12. Rainer, J. D., and Altshuler, K.Z. (Eds.): Psychiatry and the Deaf. Social and Rehabilitation Service, Department of Health, Education and Welfare, 1968.
13. Altshuler, K. Z., and Rainer, J. D. (Eds.): Mental Health and the Deaf: Approaches and Prospects. Social and Rehabilitation Service, Department of Health, Education and Welfare, 1970.
14. Rainer, J. D.: Psychiatric Services for the Deaf: Some Unmet Needs. J. Rehab. Deaf 3(1):82-89, 1969.

A City-Wide, Community-Based Aftercare Program

by Phil Reidda, Ph.D., and Thomas F. McGee, Ph.D.

In his now famous message to the Congress of the United States on mental health, President John F. Kennedy stated that "the cold mercy of custodial care would be replaced by the open warmth of community concern and capability." Central to this portion of the president's message was the thought that the number of patients receiving only custodial care in a distant institution, frequently a state hospital, could be treated in a community mental health setting near their home, and subsequently maintained in the community.

Recently, Stubblebine and Decker[1] have clearly demonstrated that community-based alternatives to psychiatric hospitalization result in a dramatic reduction in the number of patients committed as mentally ill to psychiatric hospitals. This study was particularly significant because it showed how this dramatic reduction affected the entire city of San Francisco. To date, there have been a number of indications which suggest that patients discharged from psychiatric hospitals can be maintained in the community if they receive some type of sustaining care, commonly called aftercare. Although there is limited evidence to support the beneficial effects of aftercare, there are no data which indicate that an aftercare program can have a dramatic effect on rates of recidivism for an entire city. In order to accomplish this effect in an urban setting, it is necessary to develop a network of innovative, community-based mental health facilities which possess a high degree of community support. In such facilities individuals who require sustained care for major emotional disorders could receive necessary treatment at a community level, be it day care, medication, group psychotherapy, milieu therapy, vocational rehabilitation, etc., or some combination of the above.

Community-Based Mental Health Aftercare Services

Municipally sponsored, community-based mental health facilities in Chicago have been in existence for approximately 14 years. At the present time the Mental Health Division of the Board of Health operates 16 community-based mental health centers with two more in the process of development. These centers provide a variety of direct and indirect mental health services for the majority of communities within the city. The mental health centers are relatively autonomous in terms of program development and orientation, and each works

211

closely with a local advisory board in all of its operations. The staff at each center consists of professionals and subprofessionals, many of whom are indigenous.[2]

As an important part of its direct services, each community-based mental health center operates an active aftercare program for patients discharged from psychiatric hospitals who reside within the community. Among treatment modalities used in these centers are group, family, individual, and activity therapies, frequently in conjunction with medication. Strong emphasis is placed on social rehabilitation of aftercare patients. Although the aftercare programs vary in breadth and orientation, they operate on a no-decline basis and are required to serve any resident of the community without financial charge. The mental health centers also attempt to maintain close liaison with psychiatric hospitals providing inpatient services for individuals from the community served by the mental health center.

When this study was undertaken, there were 15 community-based mental health centers in full operation. The study was designed to examine overall effectiveness of various aftercare services on a city-wide level, regardless of the particular treatment modality utilized, in relation to recidivism rates of individuals referred to the 15 individual centers.

Background

Recognition that the state hospital system is inadequate to meet mental health problems effectively has led to an intensive examination of the hospitalization and rehospitalization rates of psychiatric patients. This fact plus the cost of psychiatric hospitalization has stimulated the establishment of a wide variety of aftercare facilities.

The use of professional judgments as an estimate of need for such services has different implications than using the potential client's own perception of need.[3] In the latter case, estimates of unmet need would be based on the number of people waiting and the length of the wait. Demand, however, is not a useful index for long-range planning because the size of the demand changes depending on the number and availability of services.[3-5] The creation of new facilities for aftercare services depends on professional judgments of need and community support of these judgments.[6]

Moreover, many individuals in need of psychosocial posthospital help do not respond to offers of help or seek available help on their own.[3,5] Some who do seek help discontinue early in the treatment process.[7] Many referred to other mental health services do not accept the referral.[8,9] As a result, there appears to be a lack of continuity of care from the state hospital to the outpatient facility which is particularly difficult to achieve when dealing with patients who are returning from a psychiatric hospital to the community in which they formerly resided. Wolkon[10] indicates that to effect a successful referral from the hospital to the community center, it is important for the center's intake worker to see the patient in the hospital at least twice before release, and to see the patient within 2 weeks following hospital discharge.

Wolkon[11] also reports that two-thirds of the patients referred from psychiatric hospitals to a posthospital social rehabilitation center did not follow the referral. Patients who did participate at the rehabilitation center appeared more dependent than those who did not participate. The major differentiating factor between participants and nonparticipants was not severity of disturbance, but an underlying dependency.

This opinion is supported by a number of other studies[8,9] which indicate that the greater the effort expended in making a referral, the greater the likelihood that the patient will appear at the receiving agency. Moreover, certain aftercare programs do seem to be effective in reducing rehospitalization rates.[12-15] These studies indicate that aftercare programs can be quite effective in reducing recidivism if they are well conceived and coordinated, if the patients are carefully referred, and if concentrated efforts are made to follow up patients who fail to participate. It is equally clear, however, that aftercare programs which attract the majority of patients eligible for participation are difficult to maintain. The effectiveness of aftercare programs can be attributed to many factors. Despite some of the inherent dilemmas, aftercare services are of prime importance in community mental health centers and constitute one clear way of justifying their existence and demonstrating their effectiveness.

Method

Subjects for the present study were 1460 patients residing in the City of Chicago discharged primarily from state inpatient psychiatric institutions and referred to one of the 15 community-based mental health centers of the Chicago Board of Health, Mental Health Division during the period from July 1, 1969, to December 31, 1969. Each of the 15 participating community mental health centers was required to record and submit a list of patients referred to the center from inpatient facilities during the designated period. This list included a history of previous hospitalizations, number of visits to the center, and a history of subsequent hospitalizations. Eighteen months was the total period of time covered, from July 1, 1969, through December 31, 1970.

The data analyzed included the number of patient visits to a center, the number of patients rehospitalized, and the number of rehospitalizations. The number of patient visits was categorized into never responded or no visits, one to four visits, and five or more visits. The number of rehospitalizations was categorized into one rehospitalization and more than one rehospitalization for each of the categories of patient visits.

Results

Table 1 presents the total number of patients referred to the 15 community-based mental health centers during the period from July 1, 1969, to December 31, 1969. Of the 1460 patients referred, 356 could not be traced. Thus, 1104 patients with known dispositions remain. Table 1 indicates that the great majority (76 percent) of aftercare patients considered in this study did make some contact with the community mental health centers to which they were referred.

Table 2 shows the distribution of patients with known dispositions categorized into those patients who were maintained in the community and those patients who were rehospitalized. The rehospitalization figures include any psychiatric hospitalization by subjects in the study during the period from July 1, 1969, to December 31, 1970.

Of those patients with known dispositions who never followed referral to the community mental health center, 67 percent had to be rehospitalized. Similar patients who appeared at the community mental health center for from one to four visits or five or more visits had to be rehospitalized at the rate of 31 percent and 30 percent, respectively. A chi-square value calculated for the three categories of visits by the two types of dispositions was statistically significant $(p < 0.001)$.

A chi-square comparison between never responded and one to four visits was statistically significant $(p < 0.001)$. A chi-square comparison between never responded and five or more visits was also statistically significant $(p < 0.001)$. A chi-square comparison between one to four visits and five or more visits was not statistically significant. In other words, significantly more individuals needed to be rehospitalized if they did not come to the community mental health center than if they came for only one visit. However, no statistically significant differences with respect to rehospitalization were found between individuals

TABLE 1

Number of Patients Referred and Number of Patients Responding to Referral to 15 Community Mental Health Centers

Number of Visits	Number of Patients Referred	Patients with Known Disposition	Number of Patients Who Could Not Be Traced	Percent of Patients with Known Disposition	Percent of Patients Who Could Not Be Traced
Never responded	354	120	234	34	66
1-4 visits	463	354	109	76	24
5 or more visits	643	630	13	98	2
Totals	1460	1104	356		

TABLE 2

*Outcome for Patients with Known Disposition Who Responded to
Community Mental Health Center Referral*

Number of Visits	Patients with Known Disposition	Number of Patients Maintained in the Community	Number of Patients Rehospitalized	Percent of Patients with Known Disposition Who Had to Be Rehospitalized
Never responded	120	40	80	67
1-4 visits	354	246	108	31
5 or more	630	439	191	30
Totals	1104	725	379	34

who came to the mental health center between one and four times, and those who came five or more times.

Table 3 shows the distribution of patients who were rehospitalized, now categorized into one rehospitalization and more than one rehospitalization. Of the 120 patients who never responded to the referral, 80, or 67 percent, were rehospitalized. Of these 80, 43 (54 percent) were rehospitalized once and 37 (46 percent) were rehospitalized more than once. Of the 354 patients who came to the mental health center between one and four times, 108, or 31 percent, were rehospitalized. Of these 108, 78 (72 percent) were rehospitalized once and 30 (28 percent) were rehospitalized more than once. Of the 630 patients who came

TABLE 3

*Rehospitalization Rates for Patients Referred to the
Community Mental Health Centers*

Number of Visits	Patients with Known Disposition	Number of Patients Rehospitalized	Number of Patients Rehospitalized Once	Number of Patients Rehospitalized More Than Once
Never responded	120	80	43	37
1-4 visits	354	108	78	30
5 or more	630	191	100	91
Totals	1104	379	221	158

to the mental health center five or more times, 191, or 30 percent, were rehospitalized. Of these 191, 100 (52 percent) were rehospitalized once and 91 (48 percent) were rehospitalized more than once.

A chi-square value calculated for the three categories of visits by the two frequencies of rehospitalization was statistically significant ($p < 0.01$). A chi-square comparison between never responded and one to four visits was statistically significant ($p < 0.01$). A chi-square comparison between never responded and five or more visits was not statistically significant. A comparison between one to four visits and five or more visits was statistically significant ($p < 0.001$). In other words, for people who never responded or came to the community mental health center for five or more visits about equal percentages had to be rehospitalized once and more than once. However, for those who came to the community mental health center for from one to four visits significantly fewer had to be rehospitalized more than one time.

Implications

The above data indicate that the majority of patients discharged from psychiatric inpatient facilities and referred to community-based outpatient facilities accept the referral and make some contact with the community mental health center. Patients who make contact with the community mental health center have a significantly greater chance of remaining in the community and avoiding rehospitalization than patients who fail to make contact with the community mental health center. It is possible that less chronic patients were those making contact with the mental health centers. From the available data, however, there were no indications in this direction. In terms of outcome, it is evident that publicly sponsored, community-based mental health facilities can provide effective follow-up care for individuals returning to the community from a psychiatric hospitalization. In part, the success of this type of facility may be attributable to the advantages of a community-based mental health service: a relatively wide variety of services are readily available, many community people are involved with the mental health facility, and the community-based mental health center may be less remote and foreign appearing than other aftercare alternatives. Attendance at a community mental health center also dramatically reduces the possibility of rapid rehospitalization. In reducing rehospitalization, the number of contacts with the mental health center does not appear to be as important as the fact that some contact is made.

This study suggests that the current tendency to plan hospital discharge with the patient at the time of admission should be expanded to include appropriate staff from the posthospital service unit which will provide aftercare. There is probably a wide range of variability in the degree of outreach exercised by different mental health centers in terms of how aggressively the center encourages the discharged patient to participate in aftercare programs. Some centers may simply make themselves known to the feeder institution; others maintain an active part in the inpatient programs becoming acquainted with hospitalized people from their community and helping the patient prepare himself for return to the community. Still other mental health centers involve the potential client in the center's services before he is discharged from the hospital as an initial part of the aftercare treatment process. In this way the mental health center can become more fully integrated with the inpatient facility, and the aftercare services begin as a part of the terminal phase of inpatient service.

Unquestionably if we are fully to implement the concept of continuity of care, the relationship between community-based outpatient mental health services and inpatient psychiatric facilities must be strengthened. If strong, carefully planned, well-organized, effective liaison relationships between inpatient and community-based outpatient facilities are developed, there is no doubt that this will improve the quality and specificity of referrals made to and from both services. Such cooperative relationships can result in more available, more effective aftercare services which are used more efficiently by the recipients of the service. It also appears that community-based mental health centers should develop more aggressive follow-up procedures for those referrals which fail to come to a community mental health center at least once following hospitalization.

Developing follow-up procedures which are effective for a particular community-based mental health center is of crucial importance in terms of making any impact on the recidivism rates for a given community. In some communities a letter or telephone call to the prospective client or his family may be effective, in others a home visit may be required, and in still others a "traveling team" of mental health workers may be needed to deliver service to the patient at home. Methods of outreach need to be developed which are not only aggressive but nontraditional, and which take cognizance of both the nature of the community and the nature of the patient's particular problems.

Acknowledgments

We wish to thank the following: Murray C. Brown, M.D., Commissioner of Health, Chicago Board of Health; Jack Zackler, M.D., Assistant Commissioner of Health, Chicago Board of Health; Edward F. King, Assistant Commissioner of Health, Chicago Board of Health; and William J. O'Brien, Chairman, Chicago Board of Health, Division of Mental Health, Citizens Advisory Board.

REFERENCES

1. Stubblebine, J. M., and Decker, J. B.: Are Urban Mental Health Centers Worth It? Amer. J. Psychiat. 127:7 (January) 1971.

2. McGee, T. F., and Wexler, S.: The Evolution of Municipally Operated, Community-Based Mental Health Services, Community Ment. Health J. (in press).
3. Gurin, G., Veroff, J., and Feld, S.: Americans View Their Mental Health: A Nationwide Interview Survey. New York, Basic Books, Inc., 1960.
4. Albee, G. W., Mental Health Manpower Trends. New York, Basic Books, Inc., 1959.
5. Srole, L., Langer, T. S., Michael, S. T., Opler, M. D., and Rennie, T. A. C.: Mental Health in the Metropolis. New York, McGraw-Hill Book Co., Inc., 1962.
6. Wolkon, G. H., and Tanaka, H. T.: Professionals' View on the Need for Psychiatric Aftercare Services. Community Ment. Health J. 1(3):262-270, 1965.
7. Levinger, G.: Continuance in Casework and Other Helping Relationships: A Review of Current Research. Social Work 5(3):40-51 (July) 1960.
8. Kogan, L. S.: The Short-Term Case in a Family Agency; Part II, Results of Study. Social Casework 38(6):296-302 (June) 1957.
9. Painicky, J. J., Anderson, D. L., Nakoa, C., and Thomas, W. T.: A Study of the Effectiveness of Referrals. Social Casework 42:494-501, 1961.
10. Wolkon, G. H.: Effecting a Continuum of Care: An Exploitation of the Crisis of Psychiatric Hospital Release, Community Ment. Health J. 4(1):63-73, 1968.
11. Wolkon, G. H.: Characteristics of Clients and Continuity of Care into the Community, Community Ment. H. J. 6(3):215-221, 1970.
12. McGee, T. F., and Racusen, F. R.: An Evaluation of Alumni Group Psychotherapy for Patients Discharged from a Group Living Program. Arch. Gen. Psychiat. (Chicago) 18:420-427, 1968.
13. Beard, J. H., Pitt, R. B., Fisher, S. H., and Goertzek, V.: Evaluating the Effectiveness of a Psychiatric Rehabilitation Program. Amer. J. Orthopsychiat. 33(4):701-712 (July) 1963.
14. Wolkon, G. H., and Tanaka, H. T.: Outcome of a Social Rehabilitation Service for Released Psychiatric Patients: A Descriptive Study, Social Work 11(2):53-61 (April) 1966.
15. Wolkon, G. H., Karmen, M., and Tanaka, H. T.: Evaluation of a Social Rehabilitative Program for Recently Released Psychiatric Patients, Technical Report 29, Mental Health Rehabilitation and Research, Inc. (Hill House), Cleveland, 1970.

The Veterans Administration as a Health Care System

by Marc J. Musser, M.D., and Benjamin B. Wells, M.D.

Much has been written and said in recent years about the need for a national health care delivery system and the extent to which the health care needs of the American people are being met by a "nonsystem." Few attempts have been made to conceptualize the structure and operational nature of an appropriate delivery system. Indeed, the current preoccupation seems to be with mechanisms of payment for services in terms of various forms of health insurance, rather than with the mechanisms for expanding and improving the capacity for delivering services.

Furthermore, means must be found in the future for providing much more than the usual medical and surgical services now available. There will be a demand for greatly extended and improved psychiatric services, which must be made more readily accessible to greater numbers. In both the general medical and psychiatric areas we shall have to concern ourselves with all the social implications of an individual's state of health or nonhealth.

Any form of universal health insurance will only accentuate the need for more effective and dependable mechanisms for the provisions of services. If a health care delivery system is the best way to accomplish this, it becomes imperative that a concept be developed as a guide to the planning and implementation of future operational efforts. For such a concept, the experience of existing operational delivery systems should provide invaluable assistance.

The Department of Medicine and Surgery of the Veterans Administration is the largest system of health care delivery in the free world, and has operated as such for 25 years. Currently, in its 166 hospitals, 202 clinics, 63 nursing homes, and 16 domiciles, its staff of some 150,000 physicians, nurses, and other health care personnel provide health services to approximately 6 million of the 28 million American war veterans. This results in more than 800,000 hospital admissions and 8 million outpatient visits each year, at a cost of approximately $2 billion annually.

Providing the highest quality health care to eligible veterans is the prime mission of the VA's Department of Medicine and Surgery. After World War II, under the leadership of General Omar Bradley, Dr. Paul Hawley, Dr. Paul Magnuson, and others, the Department realized that the best way to fulfill this mission was to develop a system considerably different from the prewar facilities often referred to as "old soldiers' homes."

In its continuing development this system has come to grips with many of the problems that the country as a whole is now confronting in the sharp and growing national health care crisis. Therefore, the Veterans Administration's health care system can be considered a demonstration project that looks to the future. It can be used in many ways as a model trying to solve national problems in the delivery of health care in the months and years to come.

In his Health Message of February 18, 1971, President Nixon explicitly called for the cooperative development by the Administrator of the Veterans Administration and the Secretary of the Department of Health, Education and Welfare of "ways in which the Veterans Administration medical care system can be used to supplement medical resources in scarcity areas." A series of other requests for actions and plans, ranging from the development of new resources of health manpower to biomedical research in general and sickle cell anemia in particular, called for by the President, also implicitly involve the Veterans Administration system. These and many activities of comparable importance are already under way in our system.

Many of the essential characteristics of a successful system for the delivery of quality care are demonstrated by the Veterans Administration's system. They are directly related to the problems of the voluntary health care system of the future. Some of these characteristics are:

1. *Easy and Convenient Access.* There is no more exasperating feature of our present national health care system than the many obscure and uncertain ways patients enter it. For example, the tacit assumption that everyone has a family physician is unrealistic in a mobile and economically disparate population in which there is an overall shortage of physicians. By contrast to the general population, approximately 90 percent of the 28 million veterans live no further than 100 miles or 2 hours from a Veterans Administration health facility.

2. *A Full Spectrum of Health Resources Must Be Available So That Care Will Be Comprehensive.* An imperative of good medical practice is that the patient can be referred easily and quickly from one service to another according to his needs. This assumes a wide variety of specialties and modalities for diagnosis, treatment, and rehabilitation. Virtually all Veterans Administration hospitals are at least comparable to any good community hospital. Many serve as medical school teaching hospitals; these are comparable to university hospitals.

3. *Emphasis on Treatment at the Earliest Stage of a Patient's Disease.* This means that the system must be oriented toward ambulatory care with more intensive and sophisticated services available on call. An overwhelming majority of patients seek medical care for minor problems, which must be placed in proper relationship to life-threatening, rare, and catastrophic illness in the total array of health services and their cost. Unfortunately, the laws under which the Veterans Administration hospitals have had to operate

produce a number of administrative anomalies that limit our ability to provide the broad ambulatory services that should be available if this concept is to be fully implemented.

4. *A System Operated at Maximum Efficiency to Assure Economic Advantages to its Consumers.* One of the best ways of getting a good cost-effectiveness ratio is to delegate some of the duties previously performed more expensively by physicians to a variety of allied health personnel. The Veterans Administration hospital system, as a centrally directed system, can and does do this and is evaluating extension of this program.

5. *Prepaid Care.* This is recognized as the most effective system by most of our political, social, and health care planners and is, in fact, the basis of the several current health care programs being proposed. The Veterans Administration's health care system is a prepaid system for veterans. Basically, the prepayment is their service in the armed forces.

The Veterans Administration's health care services have always remained substantially below the cost of similar services in the private sector. The system is able to obtain expensive equipment and scarce manpower and to use them economically and efficiently. Not only can it develop and test new mechanisms for the delivery of health services, but within its hospitals and clinics, VA can and does conduct cooperative clinical and basic biomedical research in collaboration with other organizations. On VA's advisory committees and consultant rosters sit highly qualified professionals in American medicine, in the allied health professions, in the basic sciences, and in health care administration.

In terms of providing access to quality medical care, the Veterans Administration's system has demonstrated that it is possible to do things that are exceedingly difficult for individual private hospitals and their related systems to accomplish separately or together. An example is regionalization, one of the most useful "working concepts" of our time. Our system has the mechanisms to achieve the necessary high level of cooperation among its hospitals to eliminate costly duplication and make maximum use of our skills and resources. This has been done in personnel, supply, fiscal procedures, and in patient records. Similar efforts are under way in patient care.

Requests already have been received to establish outreach clinics in some of the more remote areas of the country—a type of neighborhood health center for the veteran patient. We are also evaluating mobile multidisciplinary treatment teams. These teams visit outlying communities on schedule and in cooperation with local health workers to assure the availability of needed services. Such teams have already been especially effective in mental health (as in Alabama) and in chronic pulmonary disease (as on Long Island). We are looking forward to extending other ambulatory services as the regionalization program expands.

The VA is directly involved in the education of some 11,000 medical students and 5000 interns and residents each year, as well as the allied health professions and supporting personnel categories, for example, physician assistants and subprofessional personnel in the nursing service.

At present, Veterans Administration's hospitals and clinics are affiliated with 80 medical schools, 51 dental schools, 287 nursing schools, 274 universities and colleges, and 84 community and junior colleges. Veterans Administration facilities also are used to provide health service training and work experience at novice levels to enrollees in federal economic opportunity and educational assistance programs. No other organization, agency, or group in the United States has access to the benefits of this array of academic associations.

During the current fiscal year about 50,000 students will participate in more than 60 categories of training in our institutions. The potential exists for expansion well beyond the size of the present program. When affiliated with university or college teaching resources, our hospitals constitute a highly suitable medium for the preparation of skilled workers in practically every category of health care. These workers will be available not only for our use, but for the health labor market of the voluntary system as well.

It is important to make clear another characteristic of the Veterans Administration's health care system which lends itself remarkably well to large-scale clinical research activities: cooperative research. Examples have been the demonstration that tuberculosis would respond to chemotherapy, studies of the effectiveness of psychotherapeutic drugs, of cancer chemotherapeutic agents, and of anticoagulants, as well as of other drugs and treatment modalities. We are continuing to expand and refine the techniques of such cooperative research.

Currently, one of the most popular proposals for controlling rising costs in medicine is for doctors to practice in groups. The Department of Medicine and Surgery for the past 25 years has used what is essentially a pattern of group practice for the delivery of its services. Our system is also designed to meet rising costs by efficient and economical use of buildings and modern equipment, including computers and electron microscopes.

The Veterans Administration has dealt longer with so-called consumer involvement than any other major health care organization. Daily, for 25 years, we have related to influential service organizations, civic groups, and their representatives in the Congress. With 28 million veterans in this country—who, with their families, constitute 48 percent of our population—we are sensitive to consumer reaction and involvement.

The following considerations look to the future:

1. A system or, more likely, a number of related systems will be adapted to health care delivery needs.
2. The system of medical care must permit a free movement of patients between institutions and ambulatory facilities so that effective care is provided at the lowest possible cost.

3. We must learn to develop and use varieties of health manpower according to basic principles long established in other industries.

4. Productivity measurements must be validated.

5. We must have a continuing and assured level of support for biomedical research.

6. Certain obvious cost-saving measures must be pursued. Area planning, the sharing of expensive resources between Federal and private systems, and elimination of unnecessary duplications are imperatives for the immediate future.

In conclusion, the concept that each individual is entitled to the best available care, irrespective of his social status, inability to pay, or any other nonmedical factor, has become deeply embedded in social policy. Our enormous systems of health insurance, Medicare, Medicaid, and other welfare programs are rapidly moving the nation toward if not a single system of health care, at least a single quality of service. The Department of Medicine and Surgery of the Veterans Administration is prepared to meet its responsibilities, and to make generally available the benefit of its unparalleled experience, in the vital effort of designing a system of quality health care for all Americans.

PART VII

THE AGED

Dynamic Psychotherapy of the Aged

by Harold Hiatt, M.D.

Psychotherapy, on a dynamic basis, models itself upon the techniques of psychoanalysis. A misconception existed for many years that only the relatively young could benefit from psychotherapeutic techniques. Yet many psychiatrists and psychoanalysts,[1-11] recording their experiences in treating older patients, have reported generally good results.

The senescent patient, like the adolescent, commonly has problems in areas of independence-dependence, self-identification, difficulty with other generations, asceticism, affective disturbances, and other problems in interpersonal relationships. Often the aging patient repeats psychologically many of the personal problems that he had as a child or adolescent. This "daCapo effect" of "playing through the chorus again" of one's earlier problems is extremely common in older persons.

Twelve women and 7 men with a median age of 65 have been followed over the past 15 years by the author in outpatient psychotherapy. The average number of psychotherapy hours once or twice weekly was 10.05, the least number being 6 and the greatest being 119.

Fourteen patients had depressive reaction and the remaining 5 were in the categories of phobic, hypochondriacal, and anxiety neuroses. Busse[12] has cited the frequency of depression and hypochondriacal patterns of psychoneurosis in the aging population. The precipitating event leading to their referral for psychotherapy was a recent death of a spouse, cited in 6 instances; retirement, or retirement of a spouse, in 6; and a physical illness of a somatopsychic nature or psychosomatic variety in the remaining 6. Drugs were prescribed for 5 patients, but drug treatment was ancilliary to psychotherapy and not a primary mode of treatment.

Transference

There are two unusual features in dealing with the transference phenomenon of those beyond 60, unlikely to be seen in younger patients. First, there is the realistic fact that the therapist is likely to be 20 to 30 years younger than the patient, which has a definite impact on the transference. Second, the patient over age 60 has accrued many more key figures in his past history than is true of the younger patient. A spouse may occupy a greater span of years than a parental figure and children, who may be all that remain of the patient's family constellation. In the "replaying of the chorus" of those growing older, the therapist should try to uncover the "infantile neurosis"; however, other significant figures than the patient's parents may have an impact on the transference which the patient reflects with his physician.[13] Many important figures in one's life are symbolic representations of parents; however, the degree of emotional investment goes through some shifts as one ages.

The transference reactions of this group of 19 patients could be divided into many categories with a good deal of overlapping. There were four main transference reactions: (1) parental transference (7 patients); (2) peer or sibling transference (6 patients); (3) son, son-in-law, or grandson transference (4 patients); (4) sexual transference (2 patients).

Parental Transference. All persons who are ill, psychologically or physically, use the defense of regression to some degree. A patient who comes for treatment is asking the authority, physician, parental figure for help in the classical sense. The physician and the patient, regardless of their chronological ages, are forming a parent-child relationship.

In many instances, the aged, because of dependency needs, endow the therapist not only with parental powers, but with omnipotent powers similar to the hero worship of some children. The older person, because of the decreasing number of interested persons in his environment, may transfer to the therapist a "Godlike" trust. Perhaps it is true that the older segment of our population was reared in a "God-fearing" era, but the intensity of their faith in the therapist is in some instances frightening.[6]

A 62-year-old man was seen initially on a medical ward of a private hospital where he was convalescing from his second myocardial infarction. He had severe weeping spells as evidence of his depression. The physical illness meant weakness to him and was a severe threat to his masculinity.

In weekly psychotherapy sessions, he essentially was asking, "Show me how to be a man!" It was as though he was saying to himself, if I try to prove my masculinity by work, I fear another coronary; if I am sexually aggressive toward my wife, she will discard me. This had, in reality, been a mature, giving, dedicated man, but he needed a father figure to give him permission emotionally to be a man.

Peer or Sibling Transference. Six of the nineteen patients developed a transference to the therapist which has been labeled "peer transference." As the alliance in therapy developed, this put the therapist in the role of a deceased spouse, a confidant, a close colleague, or a sibling. It is true that a peer transference did not exclude a dependent, parental, or even sexual transference. But this group looked to the therapist to confirm ego reality, to help with decision making, and to share experiences of an interpersonal nature involving other members of the family. It may be somewhat startling to the therapist to have his age ignored and be transformed into a most trusted symbol of the patient's spouse, business associate, or roommate. It is felt that this type of transference reaction is unusual in psychotherapy with other age groups.

A 71-year-old widow gave as her main complaint, "My husband dropped dead right in front of my eyes." With the husband's precipitous death, the patient was left with a large amount of money, a large suburban home, and a large amount of guilt. In weekly psychotherapy, the transference was one in which the therapist was the all-powerful referee. He was to interpret and to advise her in many areas: medical problems with her internist needed to be more clearly understood; moving from a large estate to an apartment had to be negotiated; discussion with her financial advisor had to be double-checked; continuing rivalries with her daughter and sister needed to be moderated; and ambivalent questions of her spiritual devotion required discussion. The therapist was awarded the position of the husband with all of his power and omnipotence.

Son, Son-in-law, Grandson Transference. Ten of the nineteen patients made frequent references to sons, sons-in-law, or nephews in their therapeutic sessions. Four of these were considered to have this type of transference predominating. In this situation, the patient may consider himself as the teacher and the therapist as the pupil, involving a denial of dependency. Meerloo[8] refers to this as a filial transference. On the other hand, the older patient may feel impotent, weak, set back by physical illness, or financially dependent on the younger generation. This creates the "reverse oedipal" situation. This term is confusing until one realizes that the aging patient is reacting to the younger therapist in the way a child reacts to an adult. Those who have not worked through their initial oedipal feelings apparently do not do well when the roles are reversed.

An 84-year-old widow was referred by an internist who pleaded that the psychiatrist "just see her once," a frequent appeal to those interested in geriatric psychiatry. One week prior to the interview, the patient made a suicide attempt, taking a bottle of belladonna barbiturate combination prescribed, in smaller doses, to ease her persistent abdominal cramping.
Transference to the therapist, on the one hand, was a clinging dependency alternating with a *"grande dame,"* intellectually superior, almost condescending position. The transference was reflected in two major themes seen in the pattern of several hours of therapy. The first was a discussion of the distant

past. She related, with authority, artistry, and magnetic charm, the culture, flavor, and historical significance of our fair city at the turn of the century. With validated accuracy, she described her late teens and early twenties in the social whirl of the horse-and-buggy, riverboat days of Cincinnati.

A second theme was a verbalization of anger, rivalry, and scathing indignation at her daughter and son-in-law, "the doctor." He was referred to frequently as a "dumb bastard" and an "ignorant son of a bitch," who had little class or culture and questionable professional ability.

Sexual Transference. Two patients formed an erotic or sexual transference to the therapist. Here again, one would describe dependent and peer elements in the relationship, but in the main, the response to therapy was not unlike the transference reaction seen in much younger, hysterical girls.

A 61-year-old widow described her phobia of leaving home or being alone. For the past 15 years, she had not left the city and maintained a coterie of servants including a chauffeur, a day maid, and a hired nighttime "baby-sitter" in an adjoining room. Rarely did she leave her apartment and then only with another person. In the seventh hour of a twice-a-week psychotherapy, the patient appeared in a bright pink coat, over a baby-blue dress with a pink fur hat. She protested that her fears were worse on the days of her appointment. When I pointed out that this might give some clue to the source of her fears, she associated as follows: "Thank God, it's a favorable sign; I wish I were 20 years younger [smiles at therapist]. This therapy is certainly expensive. Doctor, I have strong sensations sometimes, like a pulling at the base of the coccyx. When I was 9 or 10, I would get into the sideboard in the kitchen and take everything out, and put everything back in, and I would get a strange sensation. In grade school, when I was on a teeter-totter, I got this strange sensation. There was a boy in school, with a big hooked nose, who smelled like fish, and he told me to look and he unzipped his fly and I got that strange sensation."

Countertransference

It behooves the therapist to have a quite clear understanding of his relationship with his own parents and grandparents before treating other people's parents.[4,5,8,10,11] Countertransference reactions of oversolicitousness, idealization, and unrealistic expectations of strength on the one hand or subtle deprecations, competitive feelings, and pity on the other are commonly related to the therapist's own parents. Sometimes, the therapist feels that the older patient should be obeyed, feared, or praised, as derived from strong remnants of his own childhood. The therapist may undermine the aging persons's self-esteem if he is too condescending or patronizing.[2]

The sexual taboo with older patients is similar to the resistance met by Freud in the discovery of infantile sexuality.[8] Grotjahn[5] said that the therapist who hopes the "old person will live beyond sin and sex, like angels, is likely not to understand one of their most important sources of conflicts, guilt, and depression."

The incidence of debilitating physical illness and death is high in the aging segment of the population. Four of these nineteen patients have died, one while therapy was in progress. Countertransference reactions to this possibility must be considered. A not uncommon response by the therapist is denial and the insistence that the patient be "healthy." This may serve to counteract wishes for their death and the therapist's guilt of surviving.[9] A frightening aspect for the therapist is the deep transference of a lonely, fearful, depressed person without opportunity to form new object relationships other than that established with the therapist.[14] Rechtschaffen[14] posed the question "Does the emphasis on supportive measures for older patients in part represent a tendency to provide a less valued form of therapy for a less valued segment of the population?"

I endeavored to create a professional, peer kind of interaction with my 19 patients; however, illogical or irrational influences on countertransference appeared. They fell into four general categories:

1. *An omnipotent or unrealistic hope, with 2 patients.* A 65-year-old married woman had a reactive depression with anxiety. She had attacks of auricular fibrillation with syncope. She was seen in 31 sessions with some improvement. However, the physical decline of her arteriosclerotic heart and brain disease prevailed over psychologic treatment. In retrospect, it was unrealistic to attempt treating this patient with psychotherapy.

2. *The countertransference of feeding one's narcissism and gaining a kind of personal pleasure or personal gratification, with 8 patients.* A 68-year-old married man complained of depression and mild compulsive rituals. He was in the process of transferring his large company to his 41-year-old son, as his father had transferred the company to him. The psychiatrist was placed in the role of "superconsultant" to examine the emotional factors involved in the "changing of the guard" of a leading industrial firm. The therapist must keep close watch on his narcissistic fantasies and be careful to delineate his limited professional role to his patient and avoid the "therapist of a tycoon" role.

3. *An unreasonable anger, desire to avoid, or distinct feeling of the work of treatment, with 3 patients.* A 60-year-old married sales manager was experiencing depression with insomnia and anxiety. After 30 years of service, he became aware aware that he would never be general manager of the company. He used the therapist's support and diagnosis to gain a leave of absence with pay for 6 months and then a premature full retirement. As a crowning blow, at 2-week intervals, he submitted to the therapist forms for liberal sickness and health benefits from four different insurance companies. I had the countertransference response of "being had" by an oral aggressive patient who was acting out a plan he had devised in his many years of administrative manipulation.

4. *The feeling of pity and sorrow for a wasted life, or sympathy rather than professional empathy, with 6 of the patients.* A 61-year-old mother of five children conceived her role in life as a progressive liberal, scholar, and teacher. While in the hospital, she developed anxiety and tension of psychotic

proportions, after a radical breast operation. Metastatic carcinoma was demonstrated in the long bones. All of her five children had joined the "freaked-out" generation through drug ingestion and nomadism. Although they had all entered good colleges, four were dropouts. One son disappeared totally. Her psychosis cleared and she convalesced with supportive hormone treatment for terminal cancer. At this point, her husband of 34 years died of a coronary occlusion and she was left alone, though still quite mobile.

Discussion

The psychological ills of the older population seem to respond well to dynamic psychotherapy. Older patients are often wise, are full of zest (if they pace their energy), and may exhibit a degree of motivation in therapy not often seen in younger patients.

REFERENCES

1. Butler, R. N.: Intensive Psychotherapy for the Hospitalized Aged. Geriatrics 15:644-653, 1960.
2. Gitelson, M.: The Emotional Problems of Elderly People. Geriatrics 3:135-150, 1948.
3. Goldfarb, A. I.: Patient-Doctor Relationship in Treatment of Aged Persons. Geriatrics 19:18-23, 1964.
4. Goldfarb, A. I., and Turner, H.: Psychotherapy of Aged Persons. II. Utilization and Effectiveness of "Brief" Therapy. Amer. J. Psychiat. 109:916-921, 1953.
5. Grotjahn, M.: Analytic Psychotherapy with the Elderly. Psychoanal. Rev. 42:419-427, 1955.
6. Kahana, R. J.: Medical Management, Psychotherapy, and Aging. J. Geriatr. Psychiat. 1:78-89, 1967.
7. Kaufman, M. R.: Old Age and Aging: The Psychoanalytic Point of View. Amer. J. Orthopsychiat. 10:73-84, 1940.
8. Meerloo, J. A. M.: Transference and Resistance in Geriatric Psychotherapy. Psychoanal. Rev. 42:72-82, 1955.
9. Peck, A.: Psychotherapy of the Aged. J. Amer. Geriat. Soc. 14:748-753, 1966.
10. Wolff, K.: Individual Psychotherapy with Geriatric Patients. Dis. Nerv. Syst. 24:688-691, 1963.
11. Zinberg, N. W.: Psychoanalytic Consideration of Aging. J. Amer. Psychoanal. Ass. 12:151-159, 1964.
12. Busse, E. W.: Geriatrics Today—An Overview. Amer. J. Psychiat. 123:1226-1233, 1967.
13. Greenson, R. R.: The Classic Psychoanalytic Approach. In: Arieti, S. (Ed.), American Handbook of Psychiatry, Vol. II. New York, Basic Books, Inc., 1959, pp. 1399-1415.
14. Rechtschaffen, A.: Psychotherapy with Geriatric Patients: A Review of the Literature. J. Geront. 14:78-83, 1953.

Public Housing for the Aged

by Robert B. Sussman, M.D., and Fannie Steinberg, M.S.W.

Buildings which are almost exclusively devoted to the elderly develop their own characteristic culture. Large numbers of people who have undergone great changes in their mode of life come to live together under one roof. Old patterns of living tend to disintegrate. The old neighborhood, the familiar landscape and routine of life are given up. Old neighbors are no longer seen; familiar shops and stores are no longer frequented; the long-standing props of social identity are weakened. Even the self image may be changed abruptly. When an older person fills out an application to move to public housing, he changes from an adult to a "senior citizen."

Without the supports of the old social organization a period of personal instability ensues. To some extent the personality must be reforged to deal with the new situation. This may be done well or badly by any given person, depending on his own background, his strengths and weaknesses, and on what social conditions he must actually face in his new home.

In most buildings for the elderly, cliques are quickly formed. Groups of people of similar ethnic and social background begin to associate with each other. These groups become quite close knit. Newcomers are not admitted unless they have a similar racial and social background. There is frequent visiting between members of the group, and mutual assistance is available in times of need. Members will clean, cook, and shop for each other, and even nurse each other when sick. There is also much gossiping and backbiting, with struggles for power within and between groups. Rumors travel quickly, and news is usually distorted. If someone is hospitalized he is soon reported to be dead. With it all, the general situation is quite supportive.

In buildings which contain various age groups, relationships between aged tenants are less intense. The local community center becomes the focal point for social activity.

Those who attend the centers organize their lives around them. Birthday parties and special activities are occasions for special grooming and dressing up in party clothes and jewelry. Actions and feelings become quite intense at such gatherings, and food, if served, reflects this. It may be grabbed and quickly swallowed, or else hidden and saved. Disputes between individuals often occur, but are easily settled. Each function is an event which evokes deep reactions.

There are those elderly who cannot make the transition to their new society.

They are often cut off from their children and have few close ties. They may be failing mentally or physically. They may have experienced the death of a spouse or sibling, which is then frequently followed by rapid deterioration. If they are not involved in the social organization of their community—do not attend the center or are not members of the clique—they do not receive support and assistance. Nor does their situation come to the attention of responsible persons until it is catastrophic.

The elderly hardly ever move out of public housing. In one New York City project for older adults, there has been a turnover in only 19 of the 240 apartments in the past 5 years. Most of the removals are due to death, institutionalization, or moving in with relatives. Requests for transfer from one project to another are frequent and most often are related to concerns about safety. Purse snatching and muggings have increased. This has seriously affected the elderly because their decreased mobility makes them easy targets. They are reluctant to leave public housing despite these hazards because of finances. All that is available to low-income elderly are slum dwellings which present less physical comfort and greater dangers. The project is the home until death for most elderly, and they are well aware of this.

The New York City Housing Authority, faced with large numbers of elderly residents, has responded by developing programs of assistance and has encouraged outside agencies to do the same. Management staff is directed to work with the elderly on a personal basis. Information and assistance are given on matters such as social security, Medicare, and Medicaid. Referrals to hospitals, clinics, and social agencies are arranged. Disputes between tenants are adjudicated. Complaints, both real and imaginary, are handled. Explanations, encouragement, and advice are given. Relatives and friends are alerted in emergencies. In time of illness, physical assistance and food supplies may be organized on a temporary basis pending instutionalization or other program of assistance, which might require several days for implementation.

Authority staff helps to develop self-held groups among the tenants. Some projects have resident caretakers. These are employees who are provided with an apartment at reduced rent in exchange for getting to know the elderly residents in the building, assisting them with minor chores on the premises, and responding to emergencies.

The Authority has also encouraged public and private agencies to develop service programs for its tenants. In many instances, the Authority has provided space, maintenance, supplies, telephone service, and some staff salaries. A number of programs have been developed. The following is a sampling of the various types that are in operation and the approaches that they use.

1. The Queensbridge Health Maintenance Service for the Elderly operates at one large project, Queensbridge Houses, which houses 1500 elderly. This

program is run by the New York City Departments of Health and Hospitals with support from the National Institute of Mental Health. A general outpatient clinic operates at the project, and preventive as well as treatment approaches are attempted. The psychiatric program is small as funds are short. Physical examinations and outpatient treatment, counseling, guidance, and assistance are offered. Cases may be referred to the backup hospital. The medical staff of the program is also on the hospital staff, and an attempt is made to have the same doctors treat the patient in or out of the hospital.

2. The Senior Community Service operates at projects in the Bronx. It was organized and started by the Community Service Society, under the name of the Senior Advisory Service, and now is operated by the Housing Authority. The Department of Labor through the National Council on Aging provides partial funding. A professional social worker trains and organizes a group of indigenous elderly to provide personal, information, and referral services for other tenants in the development. The workers are paid on an hourly basis and work 20 hours per week. Information and assistance is given to help people fill out forms, contact appropriate medical and social welfare agencies, and deal with various other problems of living.

3. A resident advisor, or concierge, has been established at one large project. His function is to get to know the tenants by making home visits, and to offer security and assistance, by being available to provide help, especially at night and in emergencies.

4. Meals on Wheels is sponsored by the Isaacs Neighborhood Center. Meals are brought to the tenant's apartment at a charge of $1.50 a day, or free when necessary. This service is for tenants who are incapacitated and cannot cook for themselves.

5. Project SERVE (Serve and Enrich Retirement by Volunteer Experience) is operated by the Community Service Society in Staten Island through a grant under the Older Americans Act. Trained professional workers recruit volunteers from among the elderly residents of housing projects. These volunteers work at local institutions and hospitals. Most volunteers are between 70 and 75 years old. They are assigned to tasks at the institutions in accordance with their interests and skills. They work with patients in occupational therapy and on the wards; they do sewing and carpentry; and they assist teachers in the classroom. The program has been successful in providing opportunities for the elderly to continue to use their skills and knowledge, as well as in providing services to patients.

Summary

Elderly people turn more and more for advice and help to whatever persons are available to them who seem to be capable and knowledgeable. Many elderly people have been maintained in their homes instead of being forced into institutions because they received sympathy and assistance.

A comprehensive program of services to the elderly is required if our public housing projects are to be homes and not merely sterile shelters from the elements.

PART VIII

CONTRIBUTIONS FROM ABROAD

Continental Therapies

by Juan J. López Ibor, M.D.

Physiochemical Therapies

At the Rome Congress of Neuropsychopharmacology, Sir Aubrey Lewis, commenting on the progress recently made in the treatment of psychosis, said that if it was left to him to choose between the new therapeutics and the old "moral" methods from the time of Pinel and Tuke, he would stay with the latter. But there is no incompatibility in using various drugs at the same time as one utilizes all the possible psychological techniques, nor ought one to forget that the moral methods of the last century have been subjected to criticism, especially by Foucault, who considered them an assault on the liberty of man.

Currently, insulin therapy has practically been abandoned in almost all continental clinics, and use of electroshock treatment has also declined extraordinarily, not because of the dangers it involves or because it is ineffective, but because it is often considered a brutal method, even though it is used everywhere only under anesthesia. Yet, in schizophrenia, the convulsive therapy acts as in depressions by cutting short the sharp outbreaks and reducing their intensity. Even if there are relapses, this therapy is often effective and cannot yet be allowed to disappear from the medical arsenal.

If by means of intramuscular injection of slowly absorbed neuroleptics given each month or month and a half, a patient can be enabled to stay with his family and even sometimes continue his work, then the success of this therapeutic form would be indubitable. As a general rule, when neuroleptics are used orally, patients complain about having to take them once or more often every day.

Depressions

Therapy of depressions went from being almost completely ineffective to giving brilliant results by means of electric shock treatment. Depression, as a

233

general rule, occurs in phases or may be cyclorhythmic. In the pure phase forms, its natural tendency is toward remission. Dedichen opposed EST for depression because follow-up 5 years later showed eventual remissions in patients who had not been treated; nevertheless, it is far better for a patient to suffer only for a few week s than for 9 or 10 months.

Tricyclic antidepressives, the first of which was imipramine, were introduced in 1957 (Kuhn). Angst and Hippius believe that the action of the antidepressives does not have any nosologic boundaries, which means that the psychopathologic symptomatology can be taken into account together with the course. However, if an organic illness coexists with depression, we must of course also employ the proper somatic therapeutics. Our experience has been that the genesis of anorexia nervosa is similar to that of depression; the successes with intensive antidepressive treatments confirm this point of view.

With respect to what Freyhan called "target symptoms," the concept that depression, inhibition, and anxiety constitute three therapeutic targets which can be overcome in diverse ways can be shown to be erroneous. Inhibited depressions are much more resistant to any kind of pharmacological therapeutics than depressions with vital sadness and anxiety. In our experience, it is not proved that tricyclic antidepressives such as desipramine have any effect on the inhibited forms of the depression but are rather like analgesics against pain. Antidepressives of the amitriptyline type have a less intensive antidepressive action than those of the imipramine type, which, on the other hand, makes them more usable in the forms of depressions with an anxious, hypochondriac, and phobic content as a transition between the depressive syndrome and the neurosis. Intravenous chlorimipramine with propericiazine added can be very effective in many chronic obsessive neuroses. Antidepressives of the tricyclic type sometimes produce confusing or hallucinatory states in the old; I have also seen them appear in some organic illnesses, as in Parkinson's disease. The presence of hallucinatory paranoid syndromes during antidepressive therapy has been interpreted by some authors as due to the awakening of a latent schizophrenia; however, as Heinrich points out, this is not nosologically specific.

My experience with the action of MAO inhibitors is that they are efficient in what I have called "anxiety thymopathies," i.e., where the depressive element is colored by intense anxiety with diverse syndrome manifestations. Some anxious psychopaths belong in this category, in which the use of MAO inhibitors offers surprising results; in my unit, we use them not only orally but some of them, such as Miamid, intravenously.

To administer MAO inhibitors soon after tricyclics may be dangerous, yet we cannot leave a patient anxious and depressed with no medication for two weeks. The problem is solved by antidepressives of the dibenzodiazepine type, which make the transition from one type of medication to the other easy. This transition may, in addition, be done much more rapidly if, simultaneous with an antidepressive of this nature, 100 mg. of chlorpromazine is added daily to the therapeutic pattern.

In 1948 Cade demonstrated the favorable effects of lithium on manic patients, and Baastrup and Schou in Scandinavia showed that, with favorable doses, the reappearance of both manic and depressive phases is prevented. When these occur, we have used intense treatment with chlorimipramine, accompanied by electroshock.

Psychotherapy

Psychotherapy is widely used in Europe, although less than in the United States. Orthodox psychoanalysis reimported from the United States after World War II is concentrated in a few large cities. In general, there is a tendency toward social concepts of human problems such as advocated by Binswanger and Boss in Switzerland and Mitcherlich, Drantigan, and Dieter Wyse in Germany. The influence of existential philosophy has also been decisive (Kierkegaard, Heidegger, Jaspers, etc.). *Logotherapy* has been fundamentally cultivated in Vienna in the group founded by Victor Frankl. Caruso, following von Gebstattel, has also recently introduced social concepts. Collaboration with the family doctor is advocated by Balint in the Tavistock Clinic of London.

Aside from technicalities, such as not fixing a definite time for each psychoanalytical session but instead maintaining a flexibility in relation to the productivity of the session, what characterizes European psychoanalysis is the affirmation that the unconscious is structured like a language and in turn structures the language. According to Lacan, between 6 and 18 months, the child, even in a state of impotence and of motor incoordination, feels in his imagination consciousness and control of his body. The imaginary unification is produced by means of the identification with the image of another being as a total form and takes place through the experience of seeing one's own image in the mirror. This "mirror state" constitutes the first sketch of the ego. The intersubjective relationship, insofar as it is marked by this mirror phase, is an imaginary relationship in which the ego constitutes itself as an "alter ego," thereby establishing an aggressive tension or erotic attraction between the two. This is related to the freudian point of view of autoerotism previous to the narcissistic phase.

According to Eysenck and others, symptoms are responses conditioned by but unadapted to the environment and in consequence are due to difficulty in the learning process. There are individual differences in conditionability, just as the circumstances of the environment have their influence. All treatment of neurotics consists in dealing with present habits as though previous historical development were irrelevant, yielding better results than with analytic psychotherapy. Since the first publications of Eysenk, behavior therapy has been extended through various countries and with different aims; especially has it been used in treating alcoholism, phobias, and criminality. In my experience, the results are not brilliant. The basic theoretical problem regarding whether that which cures the symptom is the interpretation or the learning also remains unsolved. Spontaneous improvement or recovery in the neurosis occurs in 60 or 70 percent as in depressions. This intermittent course of neuroses is precisely what obscures the problems of judgment of the various treatments employed.

Psychiatric Liaisons in Czecho-slovakia, Bulgaria, Turkey, Greece, and Yugoslavia*

by Jules H. Masserman, M.D.

Following a successful series of joint meetings with various psychiatric societies in Russia, Hungary, and Yugoslavia in the autumn of 1970, the American Association for Social Psychiatry planned a tour of other Eastern European countries to further the professional exchange of information and the establishment of international friendships. Herewith a brief report of items of cultural, political, and scientific interest.

Czechoslovakia

Considerable delays and difficulties were encountered before the Czecho-slovak Ministry of Health approved our proposed joint meeting with the *National Medical Society, J. E. Purkyne,* and then only if we were designated as the International Association of Social Psychiatry rather than only its American division—possibly as an expression of residual resentment in Czech political circles over the fact that our government neither returned the Czech gold reserves we confiscated during World War II, nor compensated them with a promised steel factory, nor had yet fulfilled other treaty commitments. However, once we arrived, we were well treated as to hotel and sight-seeing accommodations by Cedok, the official tourist agency, and with unfailing hospitality by our Czech hosts.

> *Prague.* Built on seven hills, each surmounted by Gothic or baroque castles and cathedrals, Czech Praha is a handsome city whose attractions are still only slightly marred by a plethora of tourist buses—filled, significantly, with well-dressed people from other parts of Czechoslovakia—and the beginnings of urban crowding and air pollution. The housing shortage is acute: one must deposit 2 years' salary (amounting to about $3800 for a worker; $4500 or more for a physician, university professor, engineer, et al.), wait 4 to 6 years, and then pay $40 a month for a two- or three-room apartment in which six or more people must expect to live. Nor are political influences negligible: A highly trained chemist we met had to depend on relatives for support because

*Portions of this report have been published as required in Volume 17, Number 1, of the *International Journal of Social Psychiatry*.

he had been denied work for 3 years owing to his identification with a liberal party faction. Result: frequent marital tensions, high divorce and falling birth rates, and a generalized restlessness in a traditionally intelligent and progressive people still seeking rational, nonviolent solutions for their economic and political problems. Yet the memories of martyrdom in a hostile world have not faded: nowhere have I heard a more eloquent, yet resigned, account of ruthless barbarism than a Czech guide's description of how Nazi troopers cold-bloodedly raped or murdered the inhabitants of Lidice—now only a memorial rose garden. Ironically, tourist buses stop at the simple arch commemorating Lidice on the way to the scenically situated but now quietly dreary spas of government-operated Karlovy Varig and Marienbad—haunted by the frayed legends of courtly Hapsburg grandeurs.

Psychiatry in Czechoslovakia. I am happy to state that my favorable impressions[3] of the scientific premise and humanitarian practices of Czech psychiatry were fully confirmed in our meetings with the Czech National Medical Society J. E. Purkyne, as arranged with the indispensable collaboration of Drs. Eugene Vencovsky, Milan Hausner, and Zolton Kucera, respectively president, chairman of psychotherapy, and secretary of the Society.

Seminar Proceedings. After welcoming addresses by the officers of the Czech Society, I was scheduled for a Presidential Address on the Principle of Uncertainty in Psychiatry, which I may summarize as follows:

> Historical and comparative surveys indicate that whenever man becomes increasingly unsure that he can adequately anticipate and control his physical, social, or metapsychologic milieu, his anxieties mount and engender deviant patterns of attempted mastery or retreat variously termed neurotic, sociopathic, or psychotic. More sophisticated insights into the Oedipus myths than those offered by Freud reveal that they epitomize not only superficial incest fears, but also more devastating uncertainties as to dependent, competitive, and other relationships among parents and children, later "identity crises" in all concerned, the *hubris* of man's aspirations after unattainable "truths," and his ultimate defiance of the Fates themselves.
>
> In a motion picture demonstration of the severely disruptive effects of this predictive-manipulative "uncertainty," experimental animals subjected to irregularly varied cues for shock avoidance or food rewards developed phobias, compulsions, aggressions, psychosomatic dysfunctions, and other behavioral aberrations analogous to those in human neuroses or psychoses; moreover, these could be prevented or ameliorated by the monitored guidance of a conspecific automaton.
>
> The clinical relevance of the uncertainty principle, in essence, is that all therapy (Greek—*therapeien,* "service") is successful only insofar as it diminishes the recipient's uncertainty as to his physical well-being, alleviates his concerns about his interpersonal securities, and fosters comforting theophilosophic beliefs.

Dr. J. Prokupek, associate professor of psychiatry, Institute for Postgraduate Education, Prague, in association with K. Dusek then reviewed the free mental care system developed by the Ministry of Health in the CSSR after World War II. This consisted of not only the institution of modern methods in mental hospital care, but the development of psychiatric wards in general hospitals, "balneologic therapy" in specially reserved sections of famous spas such as Carlsbad, and outpatient clinics; day or night hospitals, however, are still comparatively rare (*vide infra*).

Dr. V. Dolezal, professor of psychiatry at Charles University, then described his follow-up studies of premedical students he had evaluated by means of special tests and interviews and reported that he had been able accurately to predict their progress in medical school and later in an astonishing 95 percent of cases.

Other presentations by James Sussex and by Czech colleagues at Charles University and the Research Institute will be reported elsewhere by Drs. John Schwab, who also read an excellent paper on social epidemiology (*vide infra*). The Czech titles and speakers were:

Recent Trends in Czechoslovak Neurology: Professor Dr. Z. Marek
Group Therapy by Simultaneous Cotherapists: Professor Dr. V. Dolezal
Trends in Social Psychiatry: Professor Dr. C. Skoda
Practical Training of Psychotherapists in Czechoslovakia: E. Urban, Ph.D., J. Skala, M.D., and J. Rubes, M.D.
Sociometry in Marxist Social Psychiatry: J. Gikler, Ph.D., V. Dolezal, M.D., and M. Hausner, M.D.
Hallucinogenic Mushrooms in Czechoslovakia: M. Semerdzieva, RnDr.
Genetic Influences of LSD: R. Sram, M.D., P. Gotz, M.D., and Z. Ludova, M.D.
Alcoholism and Drug Dependence in the CSSR: J. Drtil, M.D.
Drug Treatment in Czechoslovakia: O. Vinar, M.D.
The Use and Abuse of Psycholeptic Drugs in Some European Countries: M. Hausner, M.D., and Dr. Hanscarl Leuner
Hypnotherapy in Czechoslovakia: S. Kratok, M.D.

Reciprocally invited by the Czech Society, members of the American contingent spoke on various topics:

J. J. Hsu, of Pontiac, Michigan, reviewed his work on the use of electroshocks (10-40 microamperes for 30 seconds) in the negative conditioning of alcoholics in office practice, producing interim aversion to drinking but as yet no equivocal permanent results.

Robert Lynch, of La Jolla, California, described what he termed the "numinous" or "peak" LSD experience cherished by "emotionally im poverished" alcoholics as unforgettably illuminating. Dr. Lynch proposed that such experiences should be legally provided whether or not they otherwise contributed to therapy. In the discussion that followed, J. Drtil, of the Alcoholism Clinic of Charles University in Prague, and others endorsed this sentiment, some advocating LSD administration as a substitute for alcohol euphoria.

In a subsequent visit to the Horni Polata Hrebenka Day Care Center near Prague we had an opportunity to confirm in at least one instance Professor Prokupek's description of the modern modes of outpatient care in Czechoslovakia. Here Drs. Hanna Janova and Eva Karen, well-trained, dedicated, and charming disciples of Professor Ferdinand Knobloch (now emigrated to Vancouver), were conducting a most attractively built and well-staffed facility that offered varied individual, group, and community therapy to all who apply, including addicts, patients discharged from mental hospitals, and others in need of any form of psychiatric or social service.

Bulgaria

Fortunately, it was possible to schedule our visit to coincide with the Third Bulgarian International Symposium on Psychiatric Rehabilitation, also serendipitously held at Slantchev Bryag ("Sunny Beach")—a pleasant resort on the sand dunes of the placid Black Sea coast. Balkantourist, the government agency, rendered superb service, and Dr. Nikola Schipkowensky, principal organizer of the Congress, and other Bulgarian colleagues were the epitome of gracious hosts.

As previously reported,[4] the Bulgars still consider themselves the most cultured of Slavs, are still grateful to their Russian allies for delivering them from Turkish and later Nazi bondage in a succession of wars, and still acclaim their rose-scented country as the most literate, prosperous, and progressive in the Soviet orbit.

Most physicians—of whom there are now more specialists than general practitioners—are on full-time government pay although a few, such as Dr. Schipkowensky, who are especially qualified are permitted to have a private consultant practice.

Skilled professionals, including physicians, earn about $100 a month, with living expenses other than for rent and food comparable to those in our country. All enterprise is still government owned and regulated, although again, some private property is permitted: e.g., a farmer who works on a state cooperative may consume or sell the products of a small plot, and a city dweller, after paying rent on an apartment for 20 years, is given full title to it. None of this modifies the fact that rarely elsewhere in the world have we met a people more avid of good music, graceful dance, strong beer, savory wine, and general high spirits—a combination of characteristics that makes most encounters with Bulgarians a recurrent delight.

The Third International Symposium on Psychiatric Rehabilitation. As previously arranged at our request, the opening plenary session on October 20 was devoted solely to speakers from European countries, among whom were the following:

J. Temkov, director of mental health of the Czechoslovak Socialist Republic (CSSR), outlined his government's provisions for all forms of psychiatric disorder through a system of interrelated state institutions, a network of community and rural clinics, and the provision of home services by nurses and social workers under the direction of physicians and psychiatrists. Another paper, submitted but not read, reported a significant rise in the statistical incidence of behavior disorders in the CSSR, but attributed the increase to improved epidemiologic methods.

Professor Nikola Schipkowensky supplemented Dr. Temkov's report by tracing Bulgarian psychiatry from its imposed Islamic orientations during the Ottoman Empire to its present enlightened state. Psychoanalysis was to be rejected as erroneous, but all other methods were admissible including drugs, group therapies, hypnosis, and when indicated, EST and possibly lobotomy. The penal code also provided that potential criminals be treated even before they commit a crime—and were to be followed clinically in outpatient facilities as a further precaution.

J. Skala, of Charles University, described the training required of Czech psychiatrists, which comprised "knowledge of the self and others [through] proficiency in psychomimetics, hypnosis, autogenic exercises, 'psycho-gymnastics,' silent rumination, dream interpretation and the practice of yoga." Classes included coeducational sessions in sylvan or beach "retreats," during which psychiatrists, physicians, psychologists, nurses, social workers, and students cultivated "group communion."

Z. Jackowiak reported that mental health care in Poland paralleled that in the CSSR, with especial emphasis on work therapy and home supervision.

Professor Leonard Zegans, of Yale University, critically reviewed freudian and other postulates of "innate aggression" and summarized evidence in favor of the view that violent behavior is a reaction to threats, whether preceived as "real" or symbolic.

Dr. Abraham Heller reported that the acceptance of mental health service programs in Denver, Colorado, had been facilitated by placing them in general hospitals, employing personnel from local ethnic groups, and providing readily available help, including medication in crisis situations. Rates of infant mortality and state hospital admissions have decreased, but the final results are still *sub judice*.

Dr. John Schwab, of the University of Florida, concluded from his extensive survey of a Florida county that the stresses of rapid social change predispose to behavior disorders, especially in females, the poor, the unmarried, the middle-aged, and minority groups, with the greatest incidence of deviance being, almost predictably, among young black males.

H. Freeman reviewed the current status of socialized medicine in the United Kingdom, which provides free care except for dental and special appliances. One in every 125 British men and twice as many women require psychiatric services, constituting 14 percent of all consultations. The greatest problems continue to be senile pyschoses, manic depressive episodes, and schizophrenia, the prognosis of none of which has been improved by drug or other therapies.

At the request of the Symposium Program Committee, I reviewed the relevance to clinical psychiatry of my biodynamic research as follows:

> Animals subjected to seemingly—though not actually—insoluble conflicts of motivation or to difficulties of adaptation to an uncertain milieu develop persistent somatic and behavioral manifestations of anxiety, phobias, compulsions, regressions, skeletomotor and organic dysfunctions, drug addiction, disturbances in sexual and social functions, and, in severe cases, depressive retardation, hallucinations, delusions, and other bizarre psychotic-like conduct. Of all techniques of therapy investigated, the following were found to be variably effective in alleviating the disordered behavior: (1) rest and change of milieu, (2) diminution of motivational stress, (3) spontaneous reexploration, (4) forced solution of the conflict, (5) association with "normal" conspecifics, (6) guided retraining and individualized reexperience, (7) drugs such as alcohol or the barbiturates that blunted or dissociated traumatic experiences, (8) cerebral electroshock, and (9) specific surgical operations on the central nervous system. However, various combinations of these procedures were differently effective, depending on both the "constitution" and life experiences of the animal. The significance of these findings with regard to the dynamics and techniques of clinical psychiatric treatment is manifest. Clinically, however, all modes of integrative, humanitarian therapy have a common aim, namely, to restore by every ethical means available man's confidences in himself, in his fellowman, and in the various philosophies and faiths essential to his serenity.

This presentation was concluded along the lines of a more extended plenary address I had reserved for Greece (*vide infra*).

The Psychiatric Dipensary in Burgas. This old but well-preserved facility provided 400 inpatient beds, elementary workshops with industrial contracts, outpatient clinics, and home services for the therapy of various forms of behavior disorder. Alcoholics were treated by apomorphine aversion, followed by disulfiram medication and family as well as individual counseling. Morphine addicts, of which there are relatively few in Bulgaria, were subjected to direct withdrawal, during which somatic symptoms were only partially relieved. EST and insulin supplemented drug therapy for psychotics. Staff physicians worked only 36 hours a week and were given extra pay because, as Dr. Temkov informed us, "work in psychiatric hospitals is still considered dangerous."

Turkey

Even though the bus ride from Sunny Beach to Istanbul may take 10 to 12 hours, it is to be recommended for the entrancing coast and mountain scenery, the casually cheerful handling of border amenities between two countries that had been enemies for half a millenium, for the evening ride through colorful Istanbul traffic, and for the climactic arrival at the Conrad Hilton Hotel overlooking the Golden Horn of the Bosporus. Tours through the magnificent mosques, palaces, and seraglios the following day were as unforgettable as promised in every guidebook, including the local ones written in a delightful form of fractured English, but other items of information picked up from local informants were equally memorable to wit:

> Ustad Isa (a pupil of Sinan, builder of the Mosque of Suleiman the Magnificent and still considered among the three greatest architects in history) designed not only the equally beautiful Blue Mosque, but also the Taj Mahal for the Mogul Shah Jahan, who wished to be buried there beside his favorite wife, Mumtaz-Mahall. After nearly four centuries all are still widely used by the faithful for the required 10 to 30 obeisances to Allah at dawn, noon, midafternoon, and sunset.
>
> No mosque in Turkey expects either support from the government or solicitations from its worshippers; instead, they finance themselves in free competition from the nominal profit of various shops they operate on their premises.
>
> The Moslems acknowledge "Our Mother Mary" and maintain her tomb near Ephesus as a shrine freely open to Christians as well as Moslems. Jesus is respected as one of the Old Testament teachers and prophets, but is regarded, with Mohammed, as altogether mortal.

Psychiatry in Turkey. After a series of lectures at the University of Ankara in 1963, I described what I had learned of Turkish psychiatry in part as follows:

> A favorite comment among the intelligentsia is that no country can jump from the thirteenth into the twentieth century in two decades, and that Turkey is no exception. Seven of ten Turks are illiterate, but there are still no schools in most villages. The population increases by 3 percent per year with few prospects of a corresponding expansion of the economy. Many Turks are intensely religious; fortunately, the latent conflicts between the Suni and Shihite sects of Muslims no longer lead to bloodshed as they still do in Pakistan and elsewhere. Yet superstitious beliefs in the power of djinns and of the evil eye are rampant: e.g., a mother may believe she can kill her child by looking at it, however fondly, unless she immediately adds "May Allah protect you [from me]." Witches who wreak harm by involving evil djinns may not themselves be punished, but their powers to cause sorrow and disease must be counteracted by charms and incantations. Few Turks, despite their traditionally low frustration tolerance, will admit to any form of emotional disturbance, whereas a plea of physical disease is culturally acceptable: an anxious Turk consults a physician for heart trouble, a depressed one for gastrointestinal disturbances. Therefore, since 70 percent of Turkish physicians are proud of being "medical specialists" and have little knowledge of psychiatry, many patients are treated long and intensively for nonexistent organic illnesses, with much secondary iatrogenic hypo-chondriasis; in fact, few are referred for psychiatric care until prolonged somatic therapy fails, or they develop *grande hystérie* (still common in Turkish hospitals) or become frankly paranoid and homicidal. Even then their fate is in the hands of only about 200 psychiatrists in all Turkey, most of whom received what training they had in hospitals remote from modern influences.

Fortunately, striking improvement has since then been achieved on all fronts. According to Prof. Dr. Ozcan Koknel, of the University of Istanbul, and other informants, to serve a population of 22 million, there are now 500 psychiatrists in Turkey, 200 of whom practice in Istanbul (population 1.5 million). Certification requires 6 months of postgraduate work in internal medicine, a year of neurology, and two and a half years of didactic and clinical instruction in psychiatry. Training as a subspecialist for children is additional.

As to addictions, Islam forbids the use of tobacco and alcohol, but cigarettes and hookahs are on sale everywhere, and drunkenness is far from unknown. Fairly strong hashish is also smoked, but our Turkish colleagues denied that much opium either leaves the country or is used locally and pointed out that the manufacture or sale of heroin is a capital offense.

The incidence of manic depressive psychoses is 1 percent, with schizophrenia at 0.1 percent. Since elementary education, including courses in mental hygiene, is now compulsory, the populace is more literate, less superstitious, and more receptive to rational counseling and medical therapy, especially in urban centers; in Istanbul alone, there are 13 psychiatric hospitals as well as numerous free clinics.

The Bakirkoy State Mental Hospital. The entire American contingent was invited to visit this institution by Dr. Faruk Bayulkem, its highly competent superintendent who had deservedly held the post for a record-setting 32 years. We were met by a marching band of elderly patients wearing the colorfully flowing uniforms of Ottoman soldiers, playing oriental wind and percussion instruments in time with the traditional Turkish military three-step. We then toured an ancient hospital of 1500 beds, of which 100 were divided between child care and neurosurgery, and all of which were kept in remarkably operational shape on a yearly budget of less than $500,000. The medical staff comprised 60 physicians who were permitted to have afternoon or evening practices to supplement their meager salaries. Patients were admitted freely whether referred by physicians, brought by police, or by voluntary request; they could then remain a few days for transient difficulties, be treated an average of 2 months for acute psychotic reactions, or stay longer as necessary or as remanded by a court order on criminal charges. Visitors were welcome at any time. In therapy, electrosleep had been discontinued as ineffective and the use of EST and drugs was diminishing. Instead all forms of physical, social, and occupational rehabilitation were employed, as a tour through gymnasiums, workshops, studios, music rooms, libraries, and other facilities amply demonstrated. We were also shown a film of an annual hospital festival planned and staged by the patients in a manner calculated to elicit the talents, skills, and latent capacities for relatedness of even the most regressed among them.

After such hospital therapy patients were referred either to their former physician or to eight public dispensaries in Istanbul and environs where their familial and industrial readjustments were supervised. Parenthetically, however, several psychiatrists in Istanbul echoed a trenchant coda: namely, that trust in the profession was being impaired by young specialists who cared less for their patients than for financial gain and social prestige.

Greece

It would be futile here to desctibe once again the connotation of aesthetic perfection and existential empathy that one feels during any visit to the Acropolis, or the sense of awe and retrospective reverence for the origin of our Western civilization when one views Mycenae, Delphi, Cos, Epidouras, Olympia, or other classic shrines; such experiences must be reserved for the quietly contemplative inspiration of everyone fortunate enough to tour Greece. Nor would it be proper for a transient visitor to comment on the current political atmosphere in that country, other than perhaps to note that many of the alert and educated young feel repressed and resentful, but for the time being helpless to effect a chance, whereas most of their elders consider themselves not only comparatively free but grateful for the peace, order, and relative prosperity of present-day Greece.

Joint Meetings with the Athenian Institute of Anthropos and the Greek Society for the Advancement of Human Relations. These meetings were arranged in collaboration with Dr. George Vassiliou, director of the Institute and indefatigable promotor of Greek social and psychiatric studies. The views presented are herewith summarized:

Vasso Vassiliou, codirector of thc Institute, again explored some of the difficulties other nationalities encounter in trying to understand what she termed the Greek subjective culture. For example, whereas an American, to preserve his self-image, would complain only to or about an enemy, a Greek, with tears if necessary, would do so only to a person he trusts, since any sympathy so engendered would raise rather than lower his self-esteem as an obviously accepted friend. So also a Greek is never "neutral": he devoutly serves all members of his in-group (including wives and children) without ever regarding this as "love"; so also, he is profoundly suspicious of everyone else without ever thinking he is being "unfair" or "paranoid." Although the Greek mother quietly rules the family, the male considers himself everywhere dominant; asked how many children he has, he will count only his sons—yet leave the responsibility for their proper upbringing to his wife. Nor can ordinary American "intelligence tests" be applied in Greece: in a recent survey by James Gorgas only 29 percent of Athenians knew there were 52 weeks in the year. Such discrepancies make it difficult for the typical American to conduct business in Greece: the more friends he makes, the more obvious are their deep-rooted differences from his accustomed cultural norms. In commenting on Dr. Vasso Vassiliou's presentation, Dr. G. Phillipopoulos questioned the concept of a specific "subjective culture" and suggested only that when Greeks give, like everyone else, they also expect to take.

Dr. C. D. Spinellis emphasized the latent ambition of every Greek male to become a great politician, scientist, soldier—anything to demonstrate his superiority publicly—and often contentiously. Professor Rassidakes then dealt with a gentler side of the Green character by pointing out that in the Greek language the same word means both "foreigner" and "welcome guest"— whether used at home or in a seminar with American colleagues.

Two Americans contributors, Dr. Walter Bromberg and Sarah Hutchison, Ed. M., presented a paper on "Mental Patterns of an Emerging Minority Group: The American Indian," the essence of which is contained in the following slightly condensed quotation:

> The American Indian wishes to maintain his individuality and his values and culture, which until recently have been [given only] romantic literary attention. More significantly, the Indian insists that his way of life has been consistent with the preservation of natural resources, and is the very opposite of, and superior to, the industrial-commercial-success orientations of the white American. Hence, the Indian is not interested in "psychologizing" or in fine logical distinctions or philosophic analyses. He places great store in intuition, nonverbal communication, and a reverential attitude towards Nature. The essence of the native American cosmogeny lies in its acceptance of spirituality, defined as common with nature and shared by men, animals, plants, wind, sun and rain. Finally, the native urbanized and nonurban Indian repudiates psychiatric analysis as meaningless since it essentially *describes* rather than *experiences* feelings.

Becky Adelson, D.S.W., and Edward T. Adelson, M.D., then described the effort they had made through supervised group meetings to enlist ward attendants at the Bronx State Hospital in a program designed (a) to open channels of communication with the professional staff, (b) to interest attendants in further training, (c) to acquaint them with the therapeutic potentials of the hospital and (d) with community resources for therapeutic follow-up, and (e) to utilize their training in establishing rapport with their patients and aiding directly in their therapy. Unfortunately, administrative economics ended the 6-month program before its favorable short-term results could be permanently evaluated.

A paper submitted by Joyce Lowinson, M.D., and John Langrod, M.A., dealt in part with occasional opposition to community mental health centers as follows:

> The establishment of addiction treatment programs has been beset with opposition, picketing, harassment, and threats. The use of zoning regulations and court injunctions has been a standard procedure in attempting to block the opening of community-based treatment centers, whether they are

drug-free therapeutic communities such as Synanon, Daytop, Phoenix, or Odyssey House, methadone maintanance clinics, or delinquency prevention centers. The following factors have played a part: dread of an increase in crime and an influx of drugs into the community; racist sentiment manifested by fears that blacks and Puerto Ricans might come into the community for treatment with their presence leading to decrease in property values; and resentment in black and Puerto Rican communities of the presence of methadone maintenance programs because methadone is viewed as a way of "substituting one addiction for another," thus establishing white control over blacks. Nevertheless, community opposition to setting up treatment centers is usually temporary, and once the center has been operating and the community fears have been alleviated, the problem is resolved. In accomplishing this the experience of the Albert Einstein College of Medicine Methadone Maintenance Treatment Program has shown that the presence of a community relations department, staffed by successful former addicts as well as indigenous community persons, can be of great assistance. Local leaders and organizations must be contacted with a view to enlisting their cooperation and in order to explain to them the benefits that an addiction treatment program would provide to their community.

Finally, in a formal presidential address to the Greek Psychiatric Society for the Advancement of Human Relations, I spoke of psychiatry and fundamental human values along these lines:

Evolving concepts of the epistemology of science indicate that even in a discipline as "exact" as physics, "objectivity" is unattainable and operational formulae become merely subjective evaluations of statistical vectors. In this sense, if a matrix analysis were made of the essentials of what men in all times, places, and cultures have deemed deserving of effort and courage, the following ultimate (Ur) values (Latin valere, worthy of valor) would emerge:

First, the pursuit of physical health, skill, and longevity with which to explore and control the material universe.

Second, the seeking for human friendships and alliances to ameliorate loneliness and promote material welfare.

Third, the aspiration toward transcendent faiths that lend hope and significance to man's otherwise meaningless existence.

In the cumulative wisdom of our language, the term health (from Anglo-Saxon hál or hōl) has three corresponding derivations: haleness, the friendly salutation "hail," and finally "holy." Again clearly indicated are the basic objectives of all medical and psychiatric therapy:

First, to restore our patients' physical well-being and creative potentials.

Concurrently, to welcome and guide them to resume warm and fruitful human companionships, and simultaneously:

To help them regain basic serenities within themselves, with their fellowmen, and with their individually adaptive social, philosophic, and theologic faiths.

As mere mortals, we can do no more.

Yugoslavia

The official tour of the American contingent terminated in Greece, leaving the Vassiliou's and a select group of Institute students to conduct Mrs. Masserman and myself on a classical tour through the Peloponnesus prior to our departure to serve as visiting professors, respectively, in medical education and psychiatry at the University of Zagreb. There Mrs. Masserman masterfully reviewed and illustrated her recently published research on modern methods for operationally testing the medical proficiency of students and practitioners without endangering patients,[6] and I gave a series of lectures and seminars, unnecessary to review here, on biodynamic concepts and their clinical applications.[7]

Some of the most fascinating experiences during our visit were arranged by Professor Vladimir Hudolin and his wife, Dr. Visnja Hudolin, both of the University of Zagreb and both perfect hosts and invaluable friends. In effect, we were invited to sit in on the group meetings of two of the scores of therapeutic clubs Dr. Hudolin had encouraged alcoholics throughout Yugoslavia to organize and operate so as to maintain the sobriety and social usefulness of their members. The techniques employed parallel those of Alcoholics Anonymous in our country: group solidarity, democratically chosen leaders, continued education through press, radio, and television, supplementary lectures and assigned readings, the rescue of recidivist members, and mutual help with familial, social, and financial problems; however, in contrast to adverse attitudes in AA, the Yugoslav clubs accepted medical and psychiatric counseling and social service supervision from Dr. Hudolin and his professional assistants.

One such club meeting I addressed briefly was at a tuberculosis hospital some 50 miles from Zagreb, where the patients discussed and partially resolved problems arising from their arrangements with attendants and visitors for clandestine traffic in liquor, the necessity of modifying the hospital's rigid schedules of isolation and rest to allow for club activities, and other such relevant issues. Another session took place in a maximum security penitentiary after the Drs. Hudolin, Mrs. Masserman, and I had walked unescorted and unconcerned through a prison yard filled with supposedly hardened criminals who merely smiled and tipped their caps. At the meeting the club carefully considered the petitions of two members who, according to the privilege granted all prisoners by Croatian law, were due for their annual 2 weeks' leave. One inmate, who had drawn a 7-year sentence for killing his 9-month-old child in a drunken rage after his common-law wife left him, asked leave to visit his sister and former wife; however, the club decided that the two women should first be consulted by a social worker to determine directly whether they would welcome his presence. Another prisoner on a 20-year sentence for two unprovoked murders who had recently shown continued aggressiveness was altogether denied an extramural visit by majority vote; instead he was to spend the time allowed within the prison walls, but be relieved of all duties and allowed marital and other privileges.

After a lecture tour of Yugoslavia a dozen years ago, I had reported its precarious political state as follows:[8]

> It is a common saying among Yugoslavs that their country is an assembly of six republics (as now subdivided by Tito), five nations (Slovenia, Croatia, Serbia, Bosnia, and Montenegro), four languages (variants of Slavic), three religions (Catholic, Orthodox, and Moslem), two alphabets (Latin and Cyrillic), and but one desire: independence—to which an observer might add: articulate independence of each of these subdivisions, at least in part, from all the others. No two districts in Yugoslavia are quite alike, and it was Tito's recognition of the necessity for acknowledging these ethnic, cultural, economic, and religious autonomies that made the Yugoslav federation possible after 11 centuries of divisive wars.

Unfortunately, the implied prognostication had been all too accurate. By the time of our recent visit, so unmistakably intense had Croatian and other nationalist movements within Yugoslavia become that, despite President Tito's current plans for a conjoint presidency and other hopefully binding constitutional revisions, it is probable that, after Tito departs the scene, Yugoslavia will disintegrate into largely autonomous smaller states, to the ultimate disadvantage of everyone. It was this regrettable prospect in an already too fractionated world that constituted one of the few shadows on a scientifically and personally rewarding tour herein inadequately reviewed.

REFERENCES

1. Masserman, J. H.: Peripatetic Social Psychiatry. Current Psychiatric Therapies, Vol. 11. New York, Grune & Stratton, Inc., pp. 198-263.
2. In 1959, I was invited by the Czech Government to represent American psychiatry at the First Czech Psychiatric Congress with International Participation, which I reported in detail as: Battlements and Bridges in the East. In: Progress in Psychotherapy, Vol. V. New York, Grune & Stratton, Inc., 1960, pp. 231-254.
3. The 1971 Annual Report of the Czech Psychiatric Institute, obtainable in English from Dr. L. Hanzlicek, director, Praha 8, Bohnice, CSSR, summarizes many excellent physiologic, psychologic, social, and therapeutic studies conducted at the Institute, Charles University, and elsewhere in Czechoslovakia.
4. After invitations in 1963 to act as visiting professor at Beirut, Ankara, Sofia, Bucharest, and Warsaw, I wrote a report entitled "The Sphere of Psychiatry" published in Current Psychiatric Therapies, Vol. 4. New York, Grune & Stratton, Inc., 1964, pp. 280-303.
5. *Ibid.,* pp. 293-294.
6. Masserman, C. M., Solomon, L. M., and Miller, G. E. (Eds.): Clinical Simulations: Selected Problems in Patient Management. New York, Appleton-Century-Crofts, 1971.
7. Recent succinct reviews will be found in Masserman, J. H.: The Biodynamic Roots of Human Behavior, Springfield, Ill., Charles C Thomas, Publisher, 1968, and in A Psychiatric Odyssey, New York, Science House, 1971.
8. Reference 2, pp. 251-252.

Index of Names

(Italicized Numbers Refer to Contributors)

Index of Subjects